THE DEATH OF THE ASYLUM

THE DEATH OF THE ASYLUM

A CRITICAL STUDY OF STATE HOSPITAL MANAGEMENT, SERVICES, AND CARE

John A. Talbott, M.D.

Professor of Psychiatry,
Cornell University Medical College

Associate Medical Director,
The Payne Whitney Psychiatry Clinic
The New York Hospital
New York City

GRUNE & STRATTON

A Subsidiary of Harcourt Brace Jovanovich, Publishers
New York   San Francisco   London

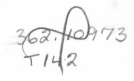

Library of Congress Cataloging in Publication Data

Talbott, John A
  The death of the asylum.

  Includes bibliographical references and index.
  1.   Psychiatric hospital care—United States.
2.   Psychiatric hospitals—United States—
Administration.   3.   Mentally ill—Care and treatment—
United States.   I.   Title.   [DNLM: 1.   Hospitals,
Public—United States.   2.   Hospitals, Psychiatric—
United States.   WM27 AA1 T14d]
RC443.T34   362.1'0973   78-12946
ISBN 0-8089-1103-1

Grune & Stratton, Inc.
111 Fifth Avenue
New York, New York 10003

Distributed in the United Kingdom by
Academic Press, Inc. (London) Ltd.
24/28 Oval Road, London NW1

Library of Congress Catalog Number 78-12946
International Standard Book Number 0-8089-1103-1

Printed in the United States of America

To the delightful and
patient women in my life

Susan, Sieglinde, and Alexandra

Contents

PART IV
SOLUTIONS

PART V
REALITY AND THE FUTURE

Acknowledgments

In this book, which addresses a single issue but which touches upon larger issues and systems continuously, I have used my background and experience in a number of different areas of psychiatry to conceptualize and discuss the problems of state mental hospitals. I have been fortunate that while most of my training and experience during my professional life has been in governmental service, I have also had a great deal of exposure to the nonprofit and university sector.

It is difficult for me to single out those individuals who should be acknowledged for their contribution in my preparation and completion of this volume since the thinking and criticism of so many were involved.

The book is the outgrowth of a series of discussions with my friend and colleague Charles Tucek, M.D., while we were both engaged in administering services in a state mental hospital in New York City. Much of the thinking in Part II—Why State Hospitals Don't Work—derives from these discussions. In addition, I owe a major debt to two groups of change agents—those who with me comprised the New York City–Long Island Regional Training Team of the New York State Department of Mental Hygiene, headed by Anita Ross, Ph.D., from 1971 to 1973, and my administrative team at Dunlop-Manhattan Psychiatric Center from 1973 to 1975. Both groups struggled with the change process in state systems, and their wisdom and collective experience provided the background for Chapter 9—The Struggle for Change. I owe a special debt to a master consultant on the change process, Jay Schulman, Ph.D., whose work with both groups was prodigious.

It was only after I left the state hospital system and returned to the university setting that I began to see many aspects of the functioning of the state mental hospital system in a clearer perspective. Of inestimable help in clarifying and developing my thinking were two seminars at Cornell University Medical College: the Administrative Problem-Solving Seminar, with Richard Berman, MBA, MPA, as well as the Seminar on the Dynamics of Administration that I have conducted for Senior Residents in Psychiatry since 1976. Both have taught me much more than I have contributed to them. While at Cornell I have had the opportunity to "pick the brains" of some of America's most prestigious group of experts in psychiatry, and I am grateful to them all, especially Jacques Quen, MD.

There are so many others to whom I am indebted: my father, John H. Talbott, MD, an extraordinary model of academic, literary, and editorial wisdom; my "educational father"—Lawrence C. Kolb, MD; my mentors in community psychiatry—Alvin Mesnikoff, MD, Matthew Parrish, MD, and Allan Elkins, MD; my models in administrative psychiatry—Stuart L. Keill, MD, Robert J. Campbell, MD, William Frosch, MD, Archie Foley, MD, and Dean W. Brooks, MD; and my "idea" people—Daniel Stern, MD, Stuart Marcus, MA, and Vivian H. Godbey, MBA, MPH.

In preparing the historical overview for this volume I was unusually fortunate in utilizing the resources of the section on the History of Psychiatry and the Behavioral Sciences, Department of Psychiatry, Cornell University Medical College, in particular Drs. Eric Carlson, Jacques M. Quen, and Norman Dain.

There are two others who have had an overriding impact on my professional and personal life and have allowed me to move in and out of systems, learning as I go. Robert Michels, MD, my current chairman at Cornell and supporter of so many of my interests and involvements over the past 15 years, has the most important trait in a friend or academic genius—the ability to criticize, to point out directions and leads to follow, and to encourage further exploration—all without the expectation of personal involvement or credit. And Susan W. Talbott, RN, MA, who has not only put up with my professional and personal wanderings through numerous fields, organizations, and systems, but who has always been so involved in the examination of the processes that it is difficult to tell where her ideas leave off and mine begin. A special word of thanks must go to the editorial department of Grune & Stratton.

And last I must thank the most energetic and dynamic secretary imaginable, Carmen Mussenden Yodbut, without whom this book would never have been written.

John A. Talbott, M.D.

Foreword

Social institutions may be created to serve human needs, but they sometimes develop into complex organisms that seem to have existences of their own. They shift from structures serving human purposes to structures that shape human lives, even becoming part of the problem for which they were designed as part of the solution. Our great public mental hospitals have become such institutions; indeed, being a patient in a state hospital is more like having a disease than receiving a treatment.

What is the problem? How has it come about? Why have previous attempts at reform failed? What are the possible strategies now? Which will work and which will fail again? What can we learn that will help us to deal with other institutions that seem to be taking over our society rather than enriching it? John Talbott addresses these questions, and many more, as he introduces us to one of the most distressing problems in the American health care system. He enlightens us about the history, sociology, economics, and politics of the state hospital system, explaining such bewildering problems as where the 350,000 patients who have disappeared from state hospitals in the last decade have gone, the difference between the theory and practice of de-institutionalization, the role of civil service unions in shaping public health programs, and why state governments ignore systems that represent the second largest item in their expense budgets. While guiding us through this complex labyrinth, Dr. Talbott never forgets what the hospitals are about—the care and treatment of mental patients.

He is eminently qualified to lead us on this journey. John Talbott is a trained psychiatrist, an experienced and practicing clinician, a former state hospital director and administrator, a former special consultant change agent, a teacher of caretakers, administrators, and consultants, a public policymaker, and, most important, a concerned human being. He has been there and has not "dropped out," but rather he has continued to press for programs and policies that will enrich the lives of the seriously, chronically, mentally ill and disabled. In this he returns to the goals that led to the first state hospitals and that have been lost in the bricks and budgets and prejudice and paper that have intervened.

Robert Michels, M.D.
Barklie McKee Henry Professor of Psychiatry and
Chairman, Department of Psychiatry,
Cornell University Medical College

THE DEATH OF
THE ASYLUM

1
Introduction: Why Be Bothered?

The publication of a book concerned with state mental hospitals coincidental with their decreasing importance in our array of mental health services may seem unnecessary. In the past decade traditional state mental institutions have virtually emptied out their masses of long-term patients—a process known by the seemingly harmless phrase of *de-institutionalization*—and newer, more flexible and ostensibly more modern services, such as community mental health centers, day hospitals, and alternative community living facilities—have been provided. Despite, or perhaps because of these developments, there is critical need at this time to focus on the state hospital or, as this institution should more appropriately be considered, the governmentally funded and operated mental hospital.

There are several cogent reasons for the examination of the operation and problems of the state mental hospital. First, there are a very large number of governmentally funded and operated mental health facilities. There are federally funded and operated Veterans Administration (VA) hospitals, most of which are primarily or importantly involved in treating the mentally ill; there are state mental hospitals, funded and operated by individual states; and there are county and municipal hospitals, which have varying responsibility for the care and treatment of the mentally ill. Second, despite the so-called "third" and "fourth" revolutions in psychiatry, the introduction of community psychiatry and psychiatric medication has not solved the problem of the chronically mentally ill, who today, because of de-institutionaliza-

1

tion, often find themselves living isolated and endangered lives in sub-standard community settings, uncared for and poorly treated. Last, examination of the state-funded and operated mental hospitals has an important bearing on the impending development of a national health insurance program that may provide comprehensive coverage of mental illness and mental disability. The care and treatment of the severely and chronically mentally ill is the largest problem, numerically, that psychiatry faces, despite the fact that to date the care of the severely and chronically mentally ill has probably had the lowest priority in the entire area of human services.

Where do we start? Several things about state hospitals are common knowledge. They are poorly staffed and inadequately funded; they occupy antiquated prisonlike buildings and house strange-looking and acting people; they are enmeshed in a bureaucratic maze of agencies, regulations, and strictures. Despite these handicaps they are expected to treat all persons who reside in the area of the state they serve; this is a clear public health responsibility. It is small wonder that, given such a responsibility without the accompanying resources to provide for each patient according to his or her needs, state hospitals fail miserably in their task.

MEDIA OUTRAGE AND PUBLIC APATHY

Since state hospitals were invented in the 1800s in this country, and invented ironically enough in response to the scandal of the mentally ill flooding the jails and poorhouses, they have been the subject of repeated exposés by the press. As one scandal seems about to be forgotten, a new one is uncovered. The public response to such exposés has been predictable. There is either a call for a new approach to the care of the mentally ill, or there is a dramatic attempt to alter an existing horror. A new approach followed the publication of Clifford W. Beers' autobiography in 1908. Although written while Beers was a patient in a private mental hospital, it focused the public's attention on all mental hospitals and was the prime mover in founding this country's "mental health movement." Cosmetic changes were made after the Willowbrook Center scandal was publicized by the press, radio, and television in the early 1970s in New York City. Even though media exposés have resulted in cosmetic changes in state hospitals or the inauguration of new facilities outside the state system, they have not produced substantial improvement in the state institutions.

No matter how scandalous the conditions, how mistreated the

patients, and how inadequate the treatment, no change can or will be made in a publicly funded institution unless there is both philosophical and financial support for such change.

Thus far this has not happened. The reasons for public apathy are numerous. First, the public continues to attach a stigma to mental illness and is prejudiced about the mentally ill, conditions that in large part are based on our own fear of our explosive inner selves and which are usually handled by putting reminders of our own frailty out of sight. Second, and coupled with the first, is the inability to identify positively and consciously with the mentally ill. Thus while people support drives against cancer or heart disease, mental illness has few crusaders. Third, there is a lack of a natural constituency for the mentally ill. The relatives of the mentally ill are hampered not only by their own stigma and prejudice, but also by whatever genetic and/or familial determinants there are to serious mental illness. Thus they themselves are not the most competent to do battle in the political/economic world. Fourth, and last, like the prison and welfare systems, the mental health system is not one with which a large number of articulate, reform-minded members of the middle class have daily exposure. There is, therefore, no constant irritant to provoke a resultant scratch. For these reasons, and others, all media scandals are doomed to failure in producing substantive change until, and unless, the attitude of the public changes.

STATE HOSPITALS AS AN EXAMPLE OF GOVERNMENTAL MEDICINE

As this country prepares to embark on a program of national health insurance, an examination of the largest single governmentally funded and operated mental health service—the state hospital—should be helpful to all who are planning for the inclusion of mental health services in a national health insurance program. The record of governmentally funded and operated mental health services has been poor. The VA system, for example, has been hampered by rigid, bureaucratic strictures, leaving it unable to deal effectively with numerous problems (most recently the Viet Nam veteran) and resulting in second-class care for long-term patients who would prefer much better care if it were available. County and municipal hospitals throughout the country are preoccupied primarily with rapid evaluation and referral to other mental health services rather than with providing effective treatment or comprehensive care themselves. The state hospitals, al-

most without exception, are anachronisms, usually only offering custodial care, and even that inadequately. For the most part the state
facilities are staffed by foreign medical graduates who are not themselves bad or incompetent, but who tend to reflect the low status of the
system.

Attempts to introduce into state hospitals professional administrators, to incorporate accountability, to initiate modern budgeting systems, and to impose quality assurance programs have usually resulted
in increased paperwork and increasingly complex bureaucratic structures rather than in improved patient care. Thus the existing care,
which is generally deplorable, too often has not improved or, in fact,
has worsened. The government attempt at reform in state hospitals is
usually addressed to the lowest level of quality, which may result in
upgrading the worst but inevitably pulls down the best by providing
new constraints to the provision of high-quality patient care.

As the reader progresses through this volume, it is imperative to
apply what is said regarding state hospitals to all government institutions delivering mental health services. The implications of the situation existing in state hospitals bears directly on all existing and future
governmentally funded and operated services. If future governmental
services resemble past state hospital care, we are in serious trouble.

PREVIEW

To examine the problems of state hospitals, this book has been
organized into five parts. Part I presents the history of state hospitals
in relation to the development of psychiatry in America. Chapter 2
starts with colonial times when patients were allowed to roam freely in
the streets or were housed in almshouses with other poor, displaced
persons. The development of mental institutions in this country, which
commonly utilized a model of moral treatment, emphasizing humane,
familial-like care in a calm secluded setting, is outlined. In the mid-
nineteenth century Dorothea Dix attempted to have the states assume
responsibility for the severely and chronically ill and argued for a
nationwide effort to build state mental hospitals. The difficulty of state
hospitals translating moral treatment into their settings, given their
population and funding, resulted in the decline of both moral treatment
and state hospitals, and a new reform movement began. This effort,
spearheaded by Clifford Beers, tried to steer efforts away from institutions toward preventive services and outpatient clinics, and coincided
with the development of newer mental health services–psychopathic
hospitals, child guidance clinics, and general hospital psychiatry.

Chapter 3 starts with the findings that emerged from World War II, namely the importance of emergency psychiatry and crisis intervention; and considers the beginnings of community mental health and the interest of the federal government in psychiatric services. Developments following World War II—such as the introduction of psychoactive drugs, the research in and development of services concerned with social psychiatry, the popularity of group therapy methods, and the introduction of social rehabilitation—made substantial changes in the practice of psychiatry. The most important was the community mental health movement, which called for an end to the massive state institutions and the movement of patients, services, and funding into community mental health centers.

Chapter 4 examines the most recent development affecting state hospitals—de-institutionalization. Dramatic drops in population occurred throughout the nation as a result of both therapeutic advances and administrative decisions to admit fewer patients and discharge many others "to the community." The latter decision was based, in part, on the availability of federal dollars for nursing home care but not for state hospital care. As a result, nursing homes now constitute the major locus for the severely and chronically mentally ill. In addition, many former mental patients have entered the welfare rolls and are housed in welfare hotels because of the lack of other housing facilities. A backlash has developed, however, and psychiatrists have become concerned with the question of whether patients are better off in bad state hospitals or wretched welfare hotels. Two results of the movement to de-institutionalize are that the difference is disappearing between the population seen in state and local hospitals and that patients now have many more admissions during their lives. The problems that de-institutionalization has exposed include (1) the difficulty of moving money from institutions to community services, (2) the inadequate range and number of community services, (3) the lack of coordination and responsibility for the severely and chronically mentally ill, and (4) the inadequacy of the state hospitals' preparation of inpatients to resume community living.

Part II provides the details of the problems that state hospitals encounter in terms of their constraints, politics, the mentalities of their staffs, and structural obstacles. Chapter 5 lists the constraints hampering state hospitals in performing their functions. These are grouped into the areas of internal (staff, patients, architecture, property, etc.), departmental (civil service, budget, legislative actions, paperwork, responsibility without adequate resources or accountability, etc), and external (judicial actions, state agencies, regulatory and accrediting bodies, the press, society, etc.).

Chapter 6 explores some of the political problems that afflict state hospitals. I suggest that psychiatrists have dealt poorly with their task of educating legislators and the public to mental health needs. As a result, inadequate attention is paid to hospital problems and funding as well as the quality of services. There are illustrations of how legislators and governors' offices utilize the scandalous conditions in state facilities for their own ends and how state facilities get caught in local/state or city/state political and economic battles.

Chapter 7 outlines the several "mentalities" of the people charged with the direction of the state hospital system. There are those who treat patient care like working in a factory, those who thrive in rigid bureaucracies and utilize its rigidity to avoid issues of patient care, those who deflect administrative attention from concern about quality to policing personnel activities, those who are preoccupied with survival instead of patient care, those whose attention is devoted to property rather than programs, those who are obsessed with numbers and quantity rather than people and quality, and finally, those whose functioning is dominated by their basic pessimism about the state hospital system.

In Chapter 8 the structural (administrative) obstacles so prevalent in state hospital systems are reviewed. Primary among these is the dilemma of being responsible for a mammoth task without the adequate resources, the commensurate authority, or the requisite accountability necessary to perform the job. There is a discussion of how budget requirements skew resources toward inpatient services instead of enabling mental health professionals to serve people in need wherever they are. Priorities are also skewed toward administrative and away from clinical duties. Additional prevalent structural attitudes are considered as well as the irrationality of the system and the problems of the low status of state facilities.

Part III represents a transition between the problems (Part II) and the proposed solutions (Part IV). It covers some of the essential elements involved in changing organizations, especially as they apply to state hospitals, as well as a summary of recent attempts to improve state mental hospitals for the better.

In Chapter 9 the change process itself is viewed from several vantage points. The reasons why state hospitals are different from other institutions are set forth. Then a typology of change affecting state hospitals is presented. This is divided into internal, external, systems, and societal changes. Although the first two changes tend to be discussed and attempted most frequently, it is the latter two that hold the most promise if meaningful improvement is to be achieved. I find 15 prerequisites for the change process to be effective, including strong support and a clear mandate from those responsible for overseeing and initiating the change and ranging from picking the right time, place, and leader to attacking on several fronts at the same time. I then give descriptions of the five fates which await change agents, some of which are totally adaptive, some personally adaptive but professionally maladaptive, and some totally maladaptive, but all of which lead eventually to leaving the system. In addition to the list of expected resistances to change, there is a basic bibliography for those interested in change in state hospitals.

In Chapter 10 the recent attempts to improve state hospitals are grouped into four categories: administrative changes, new roles for hospitals, staff development, and system changes. Administrative changes include such developments as decentralization, geographic responsibility, unitization, and the introduction of modern management techniques. In regard to assuming new roles, the state hospitals have responded either by narrowing their services (e.g., restricting admissions of the elderly) or by broadening them (e.g., offering services to alcoholics or establishing a quasi-community mental health center). In addition, some state facilities have assumed the responsibility for a range of new programs, such as inpatient, transitional, aftercare, and community services. Staff development efforts have included the initiation of the "team approach," training activities, and the opening of staff privileges to outside practitioners. The most promising recent development, which has just begun to be implemented, involves more sweeping changes in the entire mental health system. Some hospitals are cooperating in joint planning efforts, division of labor between facilities, coordination of services, and statewide unification of all mental health services.

Part IV considers several solutions for the state hospitals' dilemma. Chapter 11 gives an overall view of the range of options or solutions available, and in Chapters 12 through 15 each proposal is discussed in detail.

Chapter 12 reviews the pros and cons of retaining the state hospitals as they are currently set up, a solution that, while disavowed by most governmental agencies, is, in fact, what many persons desire and many states by their absence of activity promote. The changes that already have occurred within the system will not allow this option to be exercised, however, and state hospitals will probably not remain for long as they are now.

In Chapter 13 the most expensive and energy-draining proposal—that is, total reform of the system—is the focus. Almost every problem and constraint keeping state facilities from fulfilling their responsibility would have to be remedied truly to reform the state hospital system. Such a solution, while preserving the system and ensuring care of the chronic mental patient, will probably not occur, however, given the vested interests of the politicians, the bureaucracies, and the professionals involved.

In Chapter 14 I propose another solution, the most pragmatic of the four options suggested, that of changing the role and functions of the state hospital. Whether this involves a division of labor by geographic narrowing, patient population narrowing, specialized functioning, or a flexible fitting into the entire mental health network of a region or catchment area, I think that role change is the solution most states and state hospitals will opt for. It preserves the *status quo*, it has the appearance of change, and it promises some hope for the severely and chronically mentally ill. I am not enthusiastic about this solution, however, because it does nothing to remedy the root causes of the poor care provided in the state system.

Chapter 15 summarizes the history and arguments for and against complete closure of state facilities. Despite the sorry fate that befell the attempt to do this in the past decade, there are meritorious arguments in its favor. Most convincing is that closure does away with the state system, whose problems may be insolvable except by death. But unless monies are transferred from state to local services, the pump primed adequately before such transfer, adequate community services provided before movement is started, adequate preparation made of the community, patients, and professionals involved, and provision made for some terminal or asylum type facility—the system will work no better this time than last.

The last section of the book, Part V, provides some guidelines for the future as well as some predictions, given the themes that are inherent in the state hospital movement. For the future to be different from the past we must grasp several essential points and adhere to them. Chapter 16 considers these points: maintaining a primary focus on the needs of the severely and chronically mentally ill rather than the state hospital system, attempting to shift the public's attitudes, awareness, and status regarding chronic mental patients, bringing about change in a way different than we have in the past, altering funding formulas and budgeting processes to facilitate better patient care, altering attitudes of persons in the system, and developing a new type of accountability as well as constituency for the chronic mental patient. For the situation to change so as to benefit both the patients and the mental health system, there must be a move toward a unified system with funding and regulation at the highest governmental level with contracting of services at the lowest (local) level, thus eliminating government from the conflict-of-interest situation of both funding and running mental health services and eliminating the massive mental health bureaucracy in favor of more provision of quality patient care.

In the last chapter of the book, Chapter 17, I summarize what to me have been the major themes running through the history of the state hospital system and how these can offer us lessons for the future of governmental medicine, especially in the field of psychiatry. I predict that either state hospitals will change their roles and adapt to the needs of communities or they will, given consumer choice, Health Medical Organization's (HMO), or a voucher system, go the way of the Dodo bird.

PART I

Historical Overview

2

The History of the
State Mental Hospital

The history of the state mental hospital in the United States is in many ways the history of American psychiatry. As such, its account and interpretation are intertwined with that of psychiatry. Most historical reports of the state hospital system bear subtle or obvious biases related to the author's view of whether the state hospital has been a constructive or detrimental element in the development of mental health services in America. For instance, historians such as Dain[1] and Quen[2] see the development of state institutions as a reasonable development, and the fact that their noble purposes have failed to be realized is felt to be insufficient cause for their universal condemnation. Not surprisingly, they also see the state facility in the context of American psychiatry and mental institutions as a totality, giving ample documentation of their precursors, rather than see them as special innovative institutions. Rothman,[3] on the other hand, sees the development of the state hospital as part of a larger political and philosophical movement to control deviants and devise asylums for such, be they criminals, orphans, or the mentally ill. He, also not surprisingly, tends to emphasize (and perhaps romanticize) the care of the mentally ill by families and communities during colonial times, emphasizing the development during the Jacksonian era of a totally new institution, the asylum, to handle the growing problem of the mentally ill within the larger framework of society at that time.

Thus, for the nonhistorian who decides to present a historical overview, the task of separating the "facts," as they are given in

13

primary sources, from their subsequent utilization in secondary sources is sometimes difficult, and the presentation of the material is not necessarily that of the historian's. As a nonhistorian, I have chosen to discuss the history of the state hospital in a way that historians would probably regard as illogical but which general readers may find clear and compartmentalized. The historical summary of the development of state hospitals has been divided into the following sections.

Colonial America—Mental Hospital Precursors
The Establishment of Mental Institutions
The Era of Moral Treatment
Dorothea Dix and the Establishment of the State Hospital
The Decline of Moral Treatment and State Hospitals
Clifford Beers and the Movement Away from Institutions

COLONIAL AMERICA—MENTAL HOSPITAL PRECURSORS

In colonial America the mentally ill were found (to say they were cared for or treated would be misleading) in a number of settings.

1. Their own or relatives' homes
2. Physicians' homes
3. Jails
4. Workhouses
5. Almshouses or poorhouses
6. Wandering freely about
7. Areas near their homes, where they had been "dumped"[1]

That care at home was the benign, loving, helpful experience that some current opponents of institutions make it out to be is questionable. Some authors, such as Rothman,[3] paint a favorable picture for this home care, but others, such as Deutsch,[4] recount horrible plans for the care of the mentally ill, for example, one plan to house an insane young man in an unheated blockhouse 5 by 7 feet in size.

Jails, workhouses, and almshouses housed quite separate populations by design, although all included some of the mentally ill. A Massachusetts statute, enacted in 1699, differentiated between rogues and vagabonds who would be set to work in jails and the idle and disorderly who were obliged to work in workhouses.[3] Almshouses, on the other hand, were designed to lodge, feed, and employ the town's needy, according to Maxmen, Tucker, and Lebow.[5] Jails and workhouses were supposed to punish, almshouses to care for. Quen[2, 6] maintains that the mentally ill who were violent and difficult to control were housed in correctional facilities, whereas others who were compliant were treated as if they were merely sane paupers. In any case, beatings and floggings were not uncommonly delivered to the mentally ill for both major and minor offenses.

Another segment of the mentally ill population was allowed to wander freely about the countryside unless they were seen as a recurrent annoyance, in which case they might be trundled off at night to some neighboring village in an attempt to relieve their present host village of responsibility. The height of such inhumanity and irresponsibility displayed toward the mentally ill is described by Deutsch, who recounts that auctions were held to sell off lunatics to the highest bidder.[4]

Whatever their location, the mentally ill were kept, housed, fed, and perhaps provided with some essential goods by their families or fellow citizens, but no form of treatment or rehabilitation was intended or delivered. As already noted, frequently there was litttle sense of responsibility for them. Their plight was acknowledged, however, in some colonies. Rothman cites the first statute in Massachusetts in 1742 mandating towns to take responsibility for those "wanting of understanding, so as to be incapable to provide for his or herself."[3]

Comment should be made concerning the concepts of mental illness during this period, since they determine the attitudes toward the mentally ill carried out in the settings containing this population. Insanity was seen in Calvinistic terms, as possession by demonic forces or punishment for sin[1] or as emergence of the animalistic nature of man—the wild beast theory.[7] Also, the religious temper of the times predicated a clear separation between those who were rogues and vagabonds deserving no mercy and good honest men, worthy of sympathy and support, who had fallen upon hard times.[3]

THE ESTABLISHMENT OF MENTAL INSTITUTIONS

The mid-eighteenth century saw the establishment of the first facilities specifically intended for the mentally ill. The first institution that provided a separate unit for the mentally ill was the Pennsylvania Hospital, established in 1752 to house and care for the poor of Philadelphia. In 1773 a facility specifically for the mentally ill opened, the "public hospital" in Williamsburg, Virginia, based on the then famous Bedlam Hospital in England. In 1821 New York Hospital's Bloomingdale Asylum, based on the York Retreat, opened. These facilities for the emotionally disturbed were similar in many ways. They tended to be run by lay administrators, with physicians in consulting roles; they were intended to provide treatment, but in reality they provided custodial care; and what was designated treatment would be considered by most modern clinicians to be barbaric, inhumane, and perhaps even sadistic.[1]

At this point in history mental illness was felt to have an organic basis, albeit there was not always a demonstrable lesion on postmortem examination. Benjamin Rush, considered the father of American psychiatry, thought that mental illness was caused by congestion of the cerebral blood vessels, and the treatment (bloodletting, low sodium diets, purges, and emetics) was specifically intended to remedy this condition.[8, 9]

Chains, beatings, extremes of temperature, and inhuman living conditions were employed both in efforts to restrain patients or to shock them back to sanity. Based on the thinking of the time, which considered the mentally ill insensitive to pain, extreme cold, and so forth, such "treatment" was not only *not* considered inhuman, it was though to be potentially helpful.[1]

THE ERA OF MORAL TREATMENT

With the institution of moral treatment or moral management at the turn of the nineteenth century, American psychiatry underwent a profound change in the treatment of the mentally ill. Under the lead of a very influential group of medical superintendents,* most of whom were the original founders of what is today the American Psychiatric Asociation, American psychiatry followed the example of Pinel in France by breaking off the chains and of Tuke in England in establishing the facilities modeled after the York Retreat. Moral treatment of the mentally ill was stressed. Such a program called for humane treatment, kindness, open wards, pleasant surroundings, no or minimal restraints, structured activity, and, above all, a familiar, if not parental, relationship between superintendent and patients, which included joint dining, walks in the countryside, etc.[1, 3] Moral treatment has been described as the first conscious attempt at milieu therapy.[5]

Hospitals, such as Friends in Philadelphia, the Hartford Retreat in Connecticut, and McLean's outside of Boston, were the first to embrace the new philosophy, and results were soon reported that led to

---

*The best known of these superintendents are Luther Bell, Amariah Brigham, Pliny Earle, Samuel Kirkbride, Issac Ray, and Samuel Woodward.

great optimism. Claims of rates of cure of recent onset cases ranged from 40 percent to 100 percent and provoked a great deal of criticism and dispute. While it is clear that the reports of an 82 percent cure rate by Woodward in 1834, and 100 percent by Galt and Awl for 1842–1843 were improbable and grossly exaggerated, Quen points out that Bockoven's recalculations of Woodward's results demonstrate an actual recovery rate of 45 percent, of whom 48 percent died without a relapse.[2, 7] There is also no doubt that, in large part, the inflated claims made also hastened the downfall and disillusionment with moral treatment.

DOROTHEA DIX AND THE ESTABLISHMENT OF THE STATE HOSPITAL

Individual states had begun to establish publicly funded state mental hospitals in the late eighteenth and early nineteenth centuries. Massachusetts and New York led the movement in the late 1820s and 1830s. It was not until the appearance of Dorothea Dix on the national scene, however, that state facilities were proposed for all states.[1] Dix in the 1840s, almost singlehandedly exposed the conditions in county poorhouses and the like. She publicized the use of iron chains and shackles, the foul atmosphere, and inhumane conditions found in the facilities housing the mentally ill. She argued that local government could not care for these people, and that the burden must be assumed by the states.[3] At one point she even proposed a plan to use over 12 million acres of undeveloped land to support a federal program for the mentally ill.

Dorothea Dix's success was awesome. By 1850 almost all of the northeastern and midwestern states supported her concept of the state-funded mental hospital, and by 1860, 28 of 33 states had at least one public mental hospital.[3] Whether this was the result of an epidemic of mental illness, as Rothman argues[3] and Quen disputes,[2] or merely an epidemic of building fever, it was a visible tribute to Miss Dix, who died in 1887.

Clearly, since moral treatment was at its height of popularity at this time, state hospitals were intended to provide the same humane, benign, and enlightened care along the warm family model proposed by its pioneers. What was to happen was the reverse. The facilities established were designed to provide asylum and were located outside large population centers. In the long run this very isolation proved to be detrimental. Likewise, restrictions on mail, family visitation, and so-

cial contact with members of the patients' home communities furthered the isolation, originally felt necessary to hasten recovery from
the stresses of nineteenth-century American life. Large physical plants
were designed supposedly to provide better patient care by permitting
a diversity of medical services, more efficient organization, and better
classification of patients. Their huge size, in fact, destroyed the family
quality sought by the original medical superintendents, imposing in its
stead the impersonal and inhumane atmosphere that was such an
anathema to moral treatment. The hospitals of this era were intended
to employ more qualified physicians and be situated in more pleasant
surroundings than county poorhouses, and here, too, they failed.[4, 5]

Within these large complexes with their large populations, one of
the features of moral treatment—the emphasis on quiet, silence, order-
liness, and regular routines—so essential to moral treatment[10] became
perverted into regimentation, control, and the maintenance of the status quo. In addition, the translation of moral treatment to these new,
and in some critical ways, different institutions resulted in a focus on
the structure of the institutions. An important committee of the now-
APA addressed itself to hospital structure and in the profession we still
refer to Kirkbride buildings.[11, 12]

THE DECLINE OF MORAL TREATMENT AND
STATE HOSPITALS

The optimism about treating mental illness, so invigorating at the
beginning of the nineteenth century, had turned to pessimism by its
end. The difficulties in translating moral treatment from its original
locations to the new asylums (state hospitals) contributed to the disillusionment with moral treatment. In addition, rather than the mentally ill
receiving prompt, effective treatment and being returned to their
homes, thus maintaining a constant population—or even a decreasing
one—the census in state hospitals continued to rise, necessitating the
construction of more and more facilities to avoid the overcrowding and
disreputable conditions now appearing.[1]

State hospitals were at an additional disadvantage. They were
unable to choose whom to admit. Some of the more fortunate private
facilities could turn away the most undesirable. Consequently, the
state institutions tended to receive the most difficult, intractable, violent, and chronic patients. Simple mathematics will show that increasing the number of chronic patients has a cumulative effect on the
composition of the resident population, which grows steadily, and

compounds an already difficult situation. Another blow to the state facilities was the unwillingness of state legislatures to support these hospitals at the same per capita level; and services, staffing, and conditions inevitably decreased in quality.[3] Overcrowding had become a major problem by the 1860s and 1870s, with no remedy in sight.[9]

Another event compounded the problems experienced by state hospitals during this period. In the latter part of the nineteenth century there was a major influx of foreign-born immigrants to the United States, and these indigent new Americans were admitted to state facilities in startlingly high numbers, in part because states financed their treatment. Native-born Americans in need of care were looked after by families and communities.[3, 5] (Native Americans were also reluctant to enter state hospitals because of their "pauper insane" taint.) The differences in the cultural, social, and ethnic composition of the staff and patients in the state facilities led to a lack of understanding and distance between the two, so different from the familiarity moral treatment encouraged.

All of these problems had an inevitable impact on the treatment programs in state facilities. Restraints were used more liberally, activities were more limited, and impersonality supplanted the personal approach. Gradually moral treatment was replaced by custodial care, and a low level of custodial care at that.

Another factor in the decline of psychiatric care was the controversy raging among asylum psychiatrists and between them and the new profession of neurology.[13] Based on political, social and ideological grounds, the battle polarized psychiatrists and neurologists. John Gray, superintendent of Utica State Hospital (New York) and editor of what is now the *American Journal of Psychiatry,* was the most powerful spokesman for the group espousing the view that the diagnosis of mental illness rested on the presence of brain lesions and intellectual impairment. On the other side, Issac Ray, the superintendent of Butler Hospital (Providence, R.I.) and powerful in his own right as a founding member of what is now the American Psychiatric Association, argued for those advocating a broader psychological conception of mental disorder. The majority of neurologists, excluded from practicing in mental asylums, entered the dispute through their newly formed American Neurological Association and a private neurological journal with attacks on asylum psychiatrists and psychiatry. Weir Mitchell, the famed neurologist and psychiatrist, in 1894 launched a pointed attack on asylum psychiatrists, criticizing their isolation from the rest of medicine, their failure to support psychiatric research, their mishandling of mental patients and mismanagement of psychiatric institutions, their lack of quality training programs, and their complacency.[14] Contributing to the polarization of the profession was the debate on the cure rates for the mentally ill, referred to in the previous section, a backlash against what Deutsch has termed the "cult of curability."[4]

In the larger American society changes were taking place. Social and political reform was declining, and as the American people became more conservative and materialistic, a new conceptual force, Social Darwinism, came to ascendency.[1] Social Darwinism was the translation of evolution and degeneracy into societal terms. Its relevance to psychiatry was its implication that mental disease and the lower classes were intertwined casually and the focus of psychiatric treatment should be the prevention of propagation by these "inferior" groups.

Another outside pressure on mental health delivery was the attack on psychiatry by the press and court system. Quen notes that the earliest reported scandal described by an ex-patient of a state hospital occurred in 1833. This person detailed "abuses, cruelties, persecutions and unjustified commitments."[13, 15] A more widely read exposé in the *Atlantic Monthly*, in 1868, which later was revealed to be a fraud, fueled fires of scandal in state hospitals.[16, 17] In addition, some charges were directed at the medical superintendents themselves, accusing them of moonlighting, living luxuriously, and running plantationlike facilities.[1]

As a result, some attempts at reform were undertaken. The Massachusetts legislature in 1885 provided for boarding out harmless patients in the community. New York passed a civil service law in 1893 to remedy the abuses of cronyism and nepotism and then passed a comprehensive mental health law in 1896 regulating the system.[9] As we shall see, these reforms did not solve the problem of the state hospital.

CLIFFORD BEERS AND THE MOVEMENT AWAY FROM INSTITUTIONS

At the end of the nineteenth century several new faces appeared on the scene who had a profound influence on the course of psychiatry in our century. Most important of these were Adolph Meyer, the distinguished Swiss neuropsychiatrist who was appointed medical superintendent of the state hospital in Worcester, Massachusetts in 1895, Sigmund Freud, who provided psychiatrists for the first time with a comprehensive psychology, and Emil Kraeplin, whose textbook of psychiatry provided the most comprehensive diagnostic system yet available to the psychiatric profession.[13]

Shortly after the turn of the twentieth century, a major psychiatric "lay" figure, Clifford Beers, came to the forefront. He was to have probably the most profound effect of all on the delivery of mental health services in twentieth century America. With the publication in 1908 of *A Mind That Found Itself*,[18] his account of his hospitalization as a mental patient, Beers began a reform movement that took shape as the National Committee for Mental Hygiene and that revolutionized psychiatry in America.[1] Beers and the committee stressed prevention through effective child-rearing practices and early detection of mental illness, both of which were institutionalized in the network of child guidance clinics that soon sprang up across America.[13, 19] In addition, the committee was effective not only in sensitizing the American public about the plight of the mentally ill but also in stimulating research and training in psychiatry. Paradoxically, although Beers own account of his hospitalization was a shocking revelation of current institutional practices, the movement he spawned resulted in no effective reformation of mental hospitals. It should be noted, though, as Dain points out, a few abuses were corrected in a few hospitals and some new facilities were built.[1]

These shifts in American psychiatric practice did not occur in isolation from the rest of American society. At this time, in response to the effects of industrialization, urbanization, and monopolization, there was a national wave of social, economic, and political reform known as Progressivism, and the move to reform mental health practice was congruent with it.[1]

Another development in the delivery of services away from the state hospital model, in addition to the child guidance movement and primary prevention, was the establishment of a new psychiatric facility —the psychopathic hospital—usually associated with a university or general hospital. These facilities, such as the Phipp's Clinic in Baltimore and the Payne Whitney Clinic in New York, were modeled on German institutions and stressed short-term observation, evaluation, and treatment of acute illness. They referred their more chronic and intractable patients to "longer-stay" facilities (e.g.,state hospitals).[4] In addition, other alternatives to the traditional state hospital were tried in this era. In 1901, "tent" treatment was instituted, albeit briefly, on Ward's Island in New York City, which freed patients from their wards and placed them in outdoor surroundings. Other innovations were a hospital-based outpatient clinic at the Pennsylvania Hospital in 1904, the cottage system of smaller specialized treatment units in 1905, and state hospital aftercare clinics in Massachusetts in 1914.[9,13,20,21]

It was in this same explosive decade (1900–1910) that internist

Joseph Pratt conducted the first group therapy, a form of treatment that was to achieve wide utilization in state hospitals up to the present day. A new specialty, psychiatric social work, was established, with the first training program opening in 1914.[20]

World War I provided data, summarized and publicized by Thomas Salmon, previously the medical director of the National Committee for Mental Hygiene, that furthered the move away from institutions for the mentally ill. Salmon discovered astounding differences in the rates of disability in French and British troops suffering from combat reactions. The British troops, withdrawn from the theatening situation developed higher rates of residual illness than the French who were housed near the enemy lines and returned as promptly as possible following treatment and rest.[22] Salmon's principles of proximity (treat them where they lie), immediacy (treat them quickly), and expectancy (expect prompt recovery) became the foundation for crisis intervention, elimination of waiting lists, and local decentralized outpatient clinics.[23]

In the period between the World Wars little occured that directly affected the state hospital movement. Probably the most influential development in American psychiatry was that of psychoanalysis, which had previously been isolated in small studylike societies but was beginning to be integrated into hospital psychiatry. The most prominent example of this was the Menninger Clinic in the 1930s.[5] Following the discovery of the spirochete in 1913 and the psychiatric sequellae of the influenza pandemic of 1917, there was heightened interest in the organic causes of mental illness. With the development of the convulsive therapies in the mid and late 1930s, state hospitals at last had a form of treatment that was easily administered, efficiently delivered, and markedly effective for certain diagnostic entitities.

REFERENCES

1. Dain N: From colonial America to bicentennial America: Two centuries of vicissitudes in the institutional care of mental patients. Bull NY Acad Med 52:1179–1196, 1976
2. Quen JM: Learning from history. Psychiatr Ann 5:15–31, 1975
3. Rothman DJ: The Discovery of the Asylum: Social Order and Disorder in the New Republic. Boston, Little Brown, 1971
4. Deutsch A: The Mentally Ill in America: A History of Their Care and Treatment from Colonial Times (ed 2). New York, Columbia University Press, 1949

5. Maxmen J, Tucker GJ, LeBow M: Rational Hospital Psychiatry: The Reactive Environment. New York, Brunner/Mazel, 1974

6. Quen J: Review of Rothman DJ (reference 3). J Psychiatr Law 2:104–122, 1974

7. Bockoven JS: Moral Treatment in American Psychiatry. New York, Springer, 1963

8. Rush B: Medical Inquiries and Observations upon the Diseases of the Mind. New York, Hafner, 1962. Originally published Philadelphia, Kimber Richardson, 1812

9. Caplan RB: Psychiatry and the Community in Nineteenth-Century America. New York, Basic Books, 1969

10. Butler Hospital: Annual Reports for 1850, 1855, and 1856. Providence, 1851, 1856, 1857

11. Kirkbride T: On the Construction, Organization, and General Arrangements of Hospitals for the Insane, with Some Remarks on Insanity and its Treatment (ed. 2). Philadelphia, 1880

12. Curwen J (ed): History of the Association of Medical Superintendentents of American Institutions for the Insane. 1875

13. Quen J: Asylum psychiatry, neurology, social work, and mental hygiene: An exploratory study in inter-professional history. J Hist Behav Sci 13:3–11, 1977

14. Mitchell SW: Address before the 50th annual meeting of the American Medico-Psychological Association, held in Philadelphia, May 16, 1894. J Nerv Ment Dis 21:413–438, 1894

15. Fuller R: An account of the imprisonment and sufferings of Robert Fuller of Cambridge. Boston, 1833

16. Davis LC: A modern lettre de cachet. Atlantic Monthly 21:588–602, 1868

17. Ray I: A modern lettre de cachet reviewed. Atlantic Monthly 22:227–243, 1868

18. Beers CW: A Mind that Found Itself (ed 5). Garden City, NY, Doubleday, 1960. Originally published in 1908.

19. Whittington HG: Psychiatry in the American Community. New York, International Universities Press, 1966

20. Hamilton SW: The History of American mental hospitals, in Hall JK et al (eds): One Hundred Years of American Psychiatry. New York, Columbia University Press, 1944

21. Grob GN: The State and the Mentally I11: A History of Worchester State Hospital in Massachusetts, 1830–1920. Chapel Hill, University of North Carolina Press, 1966

22. Salmon TW: War neuroses: "Shell shock." Mil Surg 41:674–693, 1917

23. Talbott JA: Community psychiatry in the army: History, practice, and applications to civilian psychiatry. JAMA 210:1233–1237, 1969

3

The State Hospital
in Modern Times

WORLD WAR II

American psychiatry underwent a radical change with the onset of World War II. The most important developments fostering this change included the startling prevalence of mental disability revealed in the process of induction of thousands of civilians into the United States armed forces, the experiences of a large number of American physicians (many not then psychiatrists) in treating combat reactions during the war, and the reports of state hospital conditions from the large number of conscientious objectors working in these settings as alternative forms of service.

The prevalence of mental illness among draftees into the armed forces was far higher than had been anticipated. While screening techniques for the military have never isolated the factors that predict who will be a good or bad soldier, screening stations throughout the country refused induction to a high percentage of young Americans in the early months of the war because of the existence of some mental disability. Soon Congress expressed concern and this large body of legislators became sensitized about the problems America faced in dealing with the mentally ill in the 1940s.

Physicians and psychiatrists who were on active duty in the military received an equally rude awakening. Not only was the prevalence of mental illness high on induction, but also in the early stages of the war the number of combat casualities related to psychiatric conditions was strikingly high. It is reported, in fact, that during one period the number of discharges due to psychiatric reasons was higher than the total number of inductions.

On the battlefield psychiatry had forgotten the lessons that Thomas Salmon and World War I had taught. Upon their rediscovery there was a marked shift in the treatment of psychiatric combat casualties. Soldiers suffering from combat conditions, then called war neurosis, were not evacuated to safe, distant military hospitals but were treated near the lines with the cardinal principles of immediacy, proximity, and expectancy. In addition, an effort was made to place psychiatrists close to the combat lines to provide easy access to them by afflicted soldiers and thus early detection, diagnosis, and treatment, as well as to promote preventive and consultative efforts where the action was. As a result, hundreds of physicians and psychiatrists became aware of the effectiveness of short-term, goal-oriented, positive-thinking, crisis-oriented treatment approaches—which in turn, resulted in lowered rates of residual symptoms.[1]

The third force emanating from the wartime period was that of the reports of the over 3000 conscientious objectors performing alternative service in state mental hospitals. As Musto has stated, their accounts of "abysmal conditions" found in these institutions had a profound impact on postwar psychiatry.[2]

The federal government's response to these developments was in marked contrast to the mood of the 1930 Depression years. Desirous of utilizing the successful psychiatric experience on the battlefield to change the disasterous conditions at home, Congress initiated planning of new mental health programs accompanied by adequate funding, an unprecedented development. The National Institute of Mental Health was established and funded at a realistic level. The Veterans Administration launched a program to build a network of hospitals throughout the country, largely to treat psychiatric casualties of the war. And Congress passed the National Mental Health Act of 1946 in an effort to translate the success of psychiatry in the war zone to civilian life. Monies were appropriated through this bill for research, training, and assistance to the states for prevention and treatment efforts.[2]

In retrospect, however, we can see that these developments and the subsequent federal initiatives, only served to widen the gulf between state hospital psychiatry and the real world. While prevention, crisis intervention, and research into mental disease was encouraged, no effect was made to confront directly the growing numbers of chronic mental patients in state hospitals. Thus, the stage was set for the development of the community mental health movement, which in large part would also not address itself to this pressing problem.

THE ERA OF PSYCHOPHARMACOLOGY

A development that directly benefited the lives of the seriously and chronically mentally ill residing in state hospitals, and perhaps the most significant development ever in the history of institutional psychiatry, was the discovery in the 1950s of effective psychopharmacological agents. Bromides, barbiturates, and other medications had been used for some time for the mentally ill. Now for the first time psychiatrists had at their disposal antipsychotic drugs that had an immediate and telling effect on serious psychiatric conditions. In 1953 chlorpromazine was discovered, soon to be followed by meprobamate, reserpine, and chloroxipide. In the 1960s lithium was administered to the mentally ill.[3] The effect of the antipsychotics was dramatic: patients who had heretofore required constant observation, seclusion, and restraints were able to function independently within the hospitals. Brill and Patton surveyed the effects after four years of chlorpromazine use in the New York State hospital system and documented the dramatic decrease in the use of seclusion following its introduction.[4]

Many patients, previously doomed to live out their lives in state institutions, recovered sufficiently to return home. Again, Brill and Patton relate that from a high point in 1955 of 93,000 patients, the hospital population in New York State declined to 89,000 by 1959. They were able to pinpoint the actual period (1955–1956) when the state hospitals turned from steadily-increasing figures to decreasing figures in hospital populations.[4]

SOCIAL PSYCHIATRY

During the 1950s several renowned American psychiatrists kindled an interest in the individual psychotherapy of psychotic (and specifically, schizophrenic) patients. The most notable of these were Frieda Fromm-Reichmann,[5] Harry Stack Sullivan,[6] and Silvano Arieti.[7] While their influence had a great impact on the private practice of psychiatry and the training of psychiatrists, it had minimal impact on the lives of state hospital patients in comparison to the developments of the field of social psychiatry.

In an interesting way the immediate future of psychiatric programs was influenced by two completely separate streams of social psychiatric work: that in Great Britiain, which was of great practical value and dated back two decades; and that in the United States, which was more conceptual and research-based and of more recent origin. The term *social psychiatry* was used by Thomas Rennie in the mid 1950s to describe the studies he and his collaborators at Cornell University Medical College were conducting into the social factors influencing mental disorders. His work, and those of his conceptual descendants (Alexander Leighton, Leo Srole, William Langner, and Bruce Dohrenwend) continue to have a major impact on American psychiatry. But, in many ways, two other studies had a more immediate impact on the provision of public psychiatric services. Stanton and Schwartz published a detailed study of a psychiatric hospital in 1954.[8] It demonstrated how crucial were the interactions between staff members as well as between staff members and patients. A few years later Hollingshead and Redlich demonstrated the marked discrepancy that existed between the types of treatment and service settings utilized by poorer patients (state hospitals, nontalking therapies) and those used by more affluent patients (private psychiatrists, individual psychotherapy) in the New Haven (Conn.) area.[9] The Cornell group's studies demonstrated the magnitude of the incidence of mental illness in America and the role of social factors in producing mental disability; the New Haven investigators pointed out the inequity of treatment provided differing socioeconomic groups; and *The Mental Hospital* highlighted the importance of staff and environmental effects on patient behavior—and thus was of immediate practical importance to the state hospital system.

The advances of psychiatric administrators in Great Britain, going back to the 1930s, only began to be applied in American public hospitals in the 1950s. Most comprehensive was the work of Joshua Bierer with the Marlborough Experiment. Bierer instituted day, night, and weekend hospitals, social clubs for inpatients, aftercare services, and a self-governed community hostel.[10] Following the Marlborough Experiment was the "open-door" movement initiated by three hospital superintendents—Duncan MacMillian, T.P. Rees, and G. McBell.[11] Finally, Maxwell Jones pioneered and then publicized his efforts at creating a therapeutic community or milieu, one in which the entire human environment surrounding each patient became a therapeutic tool.[12] The importance of the surrounding milieu on the hospital patient was underscored by John Cummings, a New York State official, in his volume *Ego and Milieu,* published in 1962.[13] His work was regarded as a policy and procedure manual in many New York State institutions.

All of these social psychiatric developments had an impact on the treatment and care provided in state facilities.[14] Unfortunately, it was often easier to implement the suggested nonhuman environmental changes in state facilities, such as informative signs on the doors of hospital rooms, than change the attitude of staff members to a therapeutic one.

GROUP THERAPY AND SOCIAL REHABILITATION

One development in state hospitals that coincided with the initiation of the therapeutic milieu was that of group therapy, group activities, and group socialization. As mentioned previously, group therapy was pioneered in the early part of the twentieth century, and had become an essential ingredient in many programs by the 1950s. By this time Moreno's psychodrama[15] was a popular therapeutic tool in mental facilities. The 1960s and 1970s experienced a proliferation of all forms of therapeutic groups. Many of the efforts since the 1950s to habilitate and rehabilitate state hospital patients depended on group work, and, as Zusman points out,[16] this may be the most effective way to shape behavior, a necessity if patients are to move from institutionalized settings into the real world.

THE COMMUNITY MENTAL HEALTH MOVEMENT

In 1953 Kenneth Appel, then the president of the American Psychiatric Association, called for an examination of state hospitals in an address.[17] Within two years Congress had enacted the Mental Health Study Act, which created a Joint Commission on Mental Illness and Health. A great deal has been written about the reasons behind the formation of the commission, and criticisms of its functioning have been made by persons holding differing points of view. Caplan, an advocate of primary preventive mental health efforts, (which reduce the incidence of mental disorders of all types), argues that the intent of the legislators was that of preventive psychiatric efforts and that the commission opted instead to address the already mentally ill adult population by reducing the size, improving the resources, and extending the services of existing mental hospitals into the community.[18] Gardener, on the other hand, implies that concern with the chronically mentally ill was behind the federal legislation and criticizes subsequent developments for failing to tackle this population.[19]

Whatever the intent of the lawmakers, it seems clear from the commission's final report, *Action for Mental Health,* that the group wished neither to perpetuate the existing mammoth mental hospital warehouses nor to direct all our mental health efforts toward preventive services.[20] Instead the commission recommended a middle position—to build no more mental hospitals over 1000 beds and to turn those existing ones that were that size into facilities caring for the chronically ill; to build a vast network of community clinics, each serving 50,000 persons; and to direct state hospital efforts away from custodial care toward active psychiatric treatment, aftercare, and rehabilitative services.

It must be remembered that between the time the Joint Commission began its work (1955) and issued its final report (1961) several influential studies had been published demonstrating the adverse effects of psychiatric hospitalization. These included Goffman's description of institutionalization in his essay on total institutions,[21] Barton's account of institutional neurosis,[22] and Gruenberg and his associates' elucidation of the social breakdown syndrome.[23] All added fuel to the fire to burn down the state hospital.

Subsequently, as described by Bertram Brown, who was privy to the process, the government moved away from the compromise position and gave something to both sides—hospital improvement monies (HIP) to the state hospital advocates and community mental health center monies (CMHC) to the community and preventive psychiatry advocates.[24] And so it was that John F. Kennedy in February 1963 called for a "bold new approach" to the problem of mental illness in America, taking the first step toward federal responsibility for this population since Dorothea Dix's land proposal 100 years before.[25] Incorporated in the CMHC Act of 1963 were clear priorities for community services. It was apparent that few state hospitals, focused and invested as they were in the chronically mentally ill and in inpatient services, could develop adequate 24-hour emergency services, partial hospital programs, and consultation and education efforts that would enable them to capture CMHC funding. In hindsight it is clear that the CMHCs, as envisioned, would not and could not replace state hospitals and take over treatment and care of the seriously and chronically mentally ill and that such centers would in some ways only aggravate the situation by continuing a two-class system of mental health care.[26]

REFERENCES

1. Talbott JA: Community psychiatry in the army: History practice, and applications to civilian psychiatry. JAMA 210:1233–1237, 1969
2. Musto DF: The community mental health center movement in historical

perspective, in Barton WE, Sanborn CJ (eds): An Assessment of the Community Mental Health Movement. Lexington, Mass., Lexington Books, 1977

3. Ayd FJ, Blackwell B: Discoveries in Biological Psychiatry. Philadelphia, Lippincott, 1970

4. Brill H, Patton RE: Analysis of population reduction in New York State mental hospitals during the first four years of large-scale therapy with psychotropic drugs. Am J Psychiatry 116:495–500, 1959

5. Fromm-Reichmann F: Principles of Intensive Psychotherapy. Chicago, University of Chicago, Press, 1950

6. Sullivan HS: The Collected Works of Harry Stack Sullivan. New York, Norton, 1964

7. Arieti S: Interpretation of Schizophrenia. New York, Brunner, 1955

8. Stanton AH, Schwartz MS: The Mental Hospital: A Study of Institutional Participation in Psychiatric Illness and Treatment. New York, Basic Books, 1954

9. Hollingshead AB, Redlich FC: Social Class and Mental Illness: A Community Study. New York, Wiley, 1958

10. Bierer J: The Marlborough experiment, in Bellak L (ed): Handbook of Community Psychiatry and Community Mental Health. New York, Grune & Stratton, 1964

11. Weston WD: Development of community psychiatry concepts, in Freedman AM, Kaplan HI Sadock BJ (eds): Comprehensive Textbook of Psychiatry, II. Baltimore, Williams & Wilkins, 1975

12. Jones M: The Therapeutic Community. New York, Basic Books, 1953

13. Cumming J, Cumming, E: Ego and Milieu: Theory and Practice of Environmental Therapy. New York, Atherton, 1962

14. Hunt RC: Ingredients of a rehabilitation program, in An Approach to the Prevention of Disability from Chronic Psychoses. New York, Milbank Memorial Fund, 1958

15. Moreno JL: Psychodrama. New York, Beacon, 1946

16. Zusman J: The philosophic basis for community and social psychiatry, in Barton, WE, Sanborn GJ (eds): An Assessment of the Community Mental Health Movement. Lexington, Mass., Lexington Books, 1977

17. Appel K: The present challenge of psychiatry. Am J Psychiatry 111:1–12, 1954

18. Caplan G: Principles of Preventive Psychiatry. New York, Basic Books, 1964

19. Gardener EA: Community mental health center movement: Learning from failure, in Barton WE, Sanborn CJ (eds): An Assessment of the Community Mental Health Movement. Lexington, Mass., Lexington Books, 1977

20. Action for Mental Health: Final Report of the Joint Commission on Mental Illness and Health. New York, Basic Books, 1961

21. Goffman E: On the characteristics of total institutions, in Goffman E: Asylums. Garden City, NY, Doubleday, 1961

22. Barton R: Institutional Neurosis. Bristol, Eng, Wright, 1959
23. Program Area Committee on Mental Health of the American Public
     Health Association: Mental Disorders: A Guide to Control Methods.
     New York, American Public Health Association, 1961
24. Brown B: Philosophy and scope of extended clinic activities, in Bindman
     AJ, Spiegel AD (eds): Perspectives in Community Mental Health. Chi-
     cago, Aldine, 1969
25. Kennedy JF: Message from the President of the United States relative to
     mental illness and mental retardation. Am J Psychiatry 120:729–737, 1964
26. Arnoff FN: Social consequences of policy toward mental illness. Science
     188:1277–1281, 1975
27. Holland BC: An evaluation of the criticisms of the community mental
     health movement, in Barton WE, Sanborn CJ (eds): An Assessment of
     the Community Health Movement. Lexington, Mass, Lexington Books,
     1977

4
De-institutionalization

The most important single development in the delivery of mental health services by state mental hospitals in recent years is that of de-institutionalization, which in the mental health field refers to the trend to move the severely and chronically mentally ill from state hospitals to community settings. This chapter will examine the development of the movement and its rationale, its definition, the backlash that has developed in recent years, the current location of the affected population, the impact on the health system, the quality-of-life issue, problems created by the trend, and solutions to these problems.

From the time of Dorothea Dix until 1972 the number of persons being cared for in state mental hospitals rose progressively. As the population of the country grew, so did the hospital population. Since there was no effective treatment for chronic mental illness, the constant influx of persons suffering their first episode of illness added to the existing residual population of chronic patients resulting in ever increasing numbers housed in hospitals. Death and remission provided some relief from this steady increase, but not enough to alter its direction. As Kramer has noted, regardless of the total population of the United States, about 1 percent of Americans are housed in institutions at any point in time.[1]

In 1955, however, the peak in this trend was reached; since then there has been a steady decrease in the state hospital census nationally as well as in individual states.[2] The initial decline of 500 in New York State in 1955 for example, can be directly attributed to the widespread utilization of phenothiazine medication in the New York State hospital system.[2] In just four years the state hospital population had decreased by 5 percent. Nationally the same trend was observed. In 1955 there were 558,992 persons in state and county hospitals throughout the country, while in 1976 there were only 193,436—a decrease of almost two-thirds in these settings.[3]

REASONS FOR THE DRAMATIC DROP IN THE HOSPITAL POPULATION

The initial turnabout in the population housed in state hospitals, as noted, was precipitated by the widespread utilization of effective anti-psychotic medications in those facilities. The community mental health movement and the enabling legislation for community mental health centers, enacted in 1963, provided added impetus to this trend. Also not to be discounted was the strong contribution of economic factors, principally the broadening of Medicaid and Medicare reimbursement to cover persons with mental illness who could be cared for in skilled nursing facilities (SNFs) and intermediate care facilities (ICFs) rather than state mental hospitals. The reduction in state hospital populations resulting from these three developments—effective medication, treatment in community settings, and funding for mental patients in nursing homes—was, in a sense, the result of changing treatment and care practices.

It is difficult to pinpoint precisely when the decrease in hospital populations became, in addition, the result of a specific and conscious administrative decision to reduce the number of hospital residents. By the early 1970s, however, de-institutionalization became public policy in many states based on a conscious administrative decision. In New York State the first documentation of such action is considered to be a 1968 memo from the New York State Department of Mental Hygiene directing state hospital directors to ascertain whether patients (especially the elderly) were in need of treatment and if it were determined that they could be treated or cared for more appropriately elsewhere, they should neither be admitted to nor retained in state facilities.[4]

The administrative decision to shift the locus of treatment and care of the chronically ill in most instances was justified as part of a new treatment philosophy emphasizing community rather than insitutional mental health services. Many psychiatrists argued that patients are treated more effectively in small, decentralized, multipurpose, multiple-service facilities near their places of residence, family, and neigh-

borhood rather than in huge, single-purpose, inpatient-oriented warehouses, far away from their homes. As many critics have pointed out,
a more realistic explanation to explain why states shifted the locus of
care was a financial one: care for patients in nursing homes was reimbursed by Medicaid, which had a federal component and a lower daily
cost, in contrast to care for patients in state hospitals, which was
totally state funded and cost considerably more.

Proponents of de-institutionalization contended that hospitals
should only be utilized for *treatment* of the mentally ill (e.g., active
intervention, which could be expected to achieve some reversal in
symptomatology and level of functioning); other health care facilities
(nursing homes, board-and-care homes, etc.) could *care* for and house
the mentally ill. Adding to the pressure and arguments to move patients
out of state mental facilities were new laws as well as judicial decisions
that provided more circumscribed definitions of commitment procedures and directives to care for the mentally ill in the least restrictive
setting.

Kramer, for many years Chief of Biometrics and Epidemiology at
the National Institute of Mental Health (NIMH), has pointed out that
the previously mentioned treatment and care practices, as well as the
administrative decisions that brought about de-institutionalization,
were seeds falling on very fertile soil.[1] He notes that several other
developments in the 1940s and 1950s contributed to the de-institutionalization trend—the increased attention to training and research, the
increasing availability of general hospital and outpatient psychiatric
facilities, and newer psychiatric treatment methods, such as psycho-
surgery, group psychotherapy and the "total-push" approach.

DEFINITION OF DE-INSTITUTIONALIZATION

At this point we are far enough into the description of de-institutionalization to consider two definitions of the phenomenon. Bertram
Brown, former director of the NIMH, has described three components
of de-institutionalization: (1) the prevention of inappropriate mental
hospital admissions through the provision of community alternatives
for treatment, (2) the release to the community of all institutional patients who have been given adequate preparation for such a change;
and (3) the establishment and maintenance of community support systems for noninstitutionalized persons receiving mental health services
in the community.[5] Leona Bachrach, the most careful student of the
phenomenon, defines de-institutionalization as (1) the eschewal of

traditional institutional settings (primarily state hospitals) for the care of the mentally ill and (2) the concurrent expansion of community-based services for the treatment of these individuals.[5] The reader will note that both these definitions are positive rather than critical ones and both hinge on what this author would consider unachieved elements—namely, the adequate preparation of the patient for his or her return to the community and the provision of adequate community support systems and services.

THE BACKLASH TO DE-INSTITUTIONALIZATION

Considering that the process of de-institutionalization has been in effect since the 1950s, it is surprising that it took so long for a backlash to appear. Perhaps this was due to our distraction by other societal developments during this period (e.g., the Vietnam war, economic cycles, etc.), perhaps to psychiatry's unbridled zeal and enthusiasm about its own potency and that of community psychiatry, or perhaps to the cumulation of a critical mass of discharged patients in the community and the problems they posed.

During the early phases of de-institutionalization, at least in New York State, mental health professionals worked hard at developing programs to care for the newly discharged patients now living in community settings. Efforts, such as those described by Shapiro, were directed at coping with the new trend rather than condemning it.[6] By 1971, however, the stress point in New York was reached, and many professionals began to express their concerns about the programs. The Bulletin of the New York State District Branches of the American Psychiatric Association published a series of critical articles entitled "Who Will Care for the Patients?"[7] This series continued for one and a half years. During this period the New York City Commission on State-City Relations issued a report on the problems posed by de-institutionalization, entitled *State Policy and the Long Term Mentally Ill: A Shuffle to Despair*,[8] and the director of psychiatry of the Department of Social Services of New York City wrote an editorial in the official journal of the American Psychiatric Association entitled "Care of the Chronically Mentally Ill—A National Disgrace."[9]

Thereafter articles critical of the policy of de-institutionalization appeared more frequently in both professional and lay publications. For instance, *Medical World News* in 1974 featured an article, "The Discharged Mental Patient: A Medical Issue Becomes a Political One,"[10] and *The New York Times* published a series on the problem, coincidental with the gubernatorial campaign of 1974.[11] These articles were essentially reports of the problems encountered. It was not until 1976 that thorough studies of de-institutionalization began to appear. Prominent among these were a 1977 report to the Congress by the staff of the General Accounting Office,[12] the Bachrach study sponsored by NIMH,[5] and a Group for the Advancement of Psychiatry analysis of the chronically mentally ill patient in the community[13]

It is somewhat ironic that during this period, conferences and meetings continued to carry titles such as Closing State Hospitals, implying a continuance of this trend, rather than Problems Created by Deinstitutionalization and Proposed Solutions, which frequently was the undertone at the meetings.

WHERE THE PATIENTS WENT

We have noted that the state hospital population decreased from a high of 558,992 in 1955 to 193,436 in 1976. What happened to the 365,556 former mental patients? A portion of this number died, most of them elderly and suffering from chronic mental illness. Others were returned to their families and communities. Today a large number of the "returnees" can be found in nursing and board-and-care homes, in "welfare" hotels, and in flophouses.

Although the total number of Americans residing in institutions has remained constant at about 1 percent of the population for the past 30 years,[1] the proportion in different types of institutions has changed dramatically—with a marked decrease in the state hospital population mirrored by a marked increase in homes for the aged and dependent. Thus, the percentages of Americans residing in these two types of institutions have replaced each other in the 20 years between 1950 and 1970. In 1950, 39 percent of institutionalized Americans were in mental hospitals and 19 percent in nursing homes, whereas 20 percent were in mental hospitals and 44 percent in nursing homes in 1970. Taking the elderly as a subgroup, Kramer found that in 1963 the split between how many were in state hospitals versus homes was 50/50, but in 1969 it was 75/25 in favor of homes for the aged.[1] Because state facilities stopped admitting patients with organic mental syndromes, there was a drop in first admissions of such persons from 40 percent to 10 percent between 1946 and 1972. In a related development, Kramer showed that homes and schools for the mentally handicapped had an 11 percent rise in population between 1950 and 1970.

What are these places like? In terms of their population, skilled nursing facilities contain a large number of mentally impaired individuals. The General Accounting Office (GAO) report,[12] utilizing a 1974 Department of Health, Education, and Welfare (HEW) survey, states that 22 percent of their population is under the age of 65, belying the commonly held assumption that nursing homes house older people. Of these nonelderly patients, 20 percent are mentally ill and 27 percent are mentally retarded. The figures for the group over 65 are equally dramatic—33 percent have organic mental syndromes and 10 percent have neuroses or psychoses. If we use Kramer's figure of 927,514 persons residing in homes for the aged and dependent in 1970[1] and extrapolate, using the HEW figures in 1974,[12] we discover that some 406,992 persons in these homes have some form of mental disability. When we recall that state mental facilities at their height contained 558,992 persons, the magnitude of this 406,992 figure becomes more understandable.

Nursing homes represent at least 29 percent of the cost of caring for the mentally ill in America as opposed to state hospital costs amounting to 26 percent.[12] The cost of this mental health care is staggering—some $4.2 billion a year! There is no federal support for patients while they are in state facilities, nor enough support for high-quality community care programs. Therefore it is no surprise that nursing homes, which do receive federal support and which assume "total responsibility" for patients (thus obviating the need for coordination of psychiatric care), have gathered such a large share of the mental health dollar.[12]

The discussion has not really answered our question, "What are these places like?" We are all aware of the widespread attention that the press has paid to the problems found in nursing homes—not just problems of fraud and mismanagement, but also those of brutality, inhumane conditions, and the lack of programs for the residents. A professional study of such facilities, conducted by the Joint Information Service of the American Psychiatric Association and the National Association for Mental Health,[14] was critical of several features of such homes: the lack of involvement of families, the placement of persons in homes when they could be in a facility a level lower, the lack of available psychiatric care, the low pay of the staff, and farce of maintaining that these homes were "in the community," which they frequently were not. On the whole, however, the study found the conditions not as shocking as commonly thought or described in the press.

The study failed to answer the question, which may be unanswerable "Is the quality of life better in such homes than in state facilities?"

THE QUALITY-OF-LIFE ISSUE

The question of where patients are better off, in state hospitals or community facilities, is central to the debate on de-institutionalization. It is difficult, if not impossible, to answer because each is represented by a wide range of types and quality of facility. There are splendid state facilities with young, well-trained staffs, competent medical leaders and lay administrators, and effective active treatment and rehabilitation programs just as there are clean, well-managed and well-staffed homes with community mental health teams providing active follow-up care. Unfortunately, there are far too many bad state hospitals and bad nursing and board-and-care homes, all of which may suffer the same deficiencies—isolation from the community, large size, decrepit buildings, inhumane or nonexistent care, and underpaid, undertrained, and inadequate staffs, who have long since given in to the despair their jobs may engender.

Thus the question posed is not answerable in absolutes. Instead, one must look at individual cases, an approach that is not favored by bureaucracies, systems, and movements, which thrive on the single answer. As Wing has stated, "Universal denunciation of any one type of setting is likely to be harmful since it is clearly not based on rational principles of assessment, treatment or care."[15] On the other hand, there are respectable studies that discredit complete systems. Lamb and Goertzel, for example, indicate that the quality of life is bad enough in both board-and-care and state hospital settings to warrant preference to be given to "other types" of living arrangements.[16]

No longer can anyone maintain that state hospitals must be emptied simply because they are "so awful"—because the settings we have allowed to replace them are just as bad as their predecessors. No, the answer lies in looking at the problem again. And the problem is *the treatment and care* of the chronic mental patient. Unless we are able to address this population and this problem, it does not matter what we call the buildings—state hospitals, community mental health centers, or nursing homes. What we must do is establish and fund adequate programs for the treatment of the chronically mentally ill. It is this approach that is most lacking in our current discussion about the merits and demerits of de-institutionalization.

**IMPACT OF DE-INSTITUTIONALIZATION ON THE
HEALTH SYSTEM**

Two major developments in the delivery of mental health care in
this country have been closely related to the process of de-institutionalization. The first is that the previous difference between the population seen in local hospitals (city, county, and voluntary) and that seen
by the state facilities has begun to disappear. In the past first admissions and acute episodes tended to be seen in local hospitals, and
chronic patients tended to be treated in state facilities. With de-institutionalization and the refusal of state facilities to admit chronic and
geriatric patients, the profiles of patients in the two systems have begun to approximate each other. To some this equalization represents a
long-awaited abolition of the two-class system of mental health care,[17]
while to others it suggests that there may be a mistake in the allocation
of scarce resources and effective utilization of facilities.[18] The magnitude of the shift in the locus of treatment of the severely and chronically mentally ill can be seen from available statistics[1] In 1955 (the year
of the greatest state hospital population) 50 percent of patient care
episodes were treated in state facilities, whereas in 1973 only 12 percent were. However, community mental health centers, not even con-
ceived in 1955, in 1973 treated 23 percent and outpatient facilities
(which accounted for 23 percent in 1955) saw 45 percent of such
patients.

The second major impact of de-institutionalization on the mental
health system concerns the phenomenon of readmission. While the
residual chronic population of state facilities decreased, total admissions continued to rise (until 1972) largely as a result of the increasing
number of readmissions. This phenomenon—more patients spending
less time per episode in a hospital but entering the hospital a greater
number of times—is what the author has described elsewhere as the
"revolving door."[19] Readmissions, which in 1969 had accounted for 47
percent of those entering state hospitals, by 1972 constituted 54 percent of all admissions. In some states the figures rose from 43 percent
in 1963 to 70 percent in 1974.[12] In some areas, such as New York City,
many professionals doubt whether any patient can be provided
prompt, effective and efficient psychiatric treatment if he or she is
treated by different facilities for either each particular episode of illness or for separate episodes.

PROBLEMS POSED BY DE-INSTITUTIONALIZATION

The most crucial problem that de-institutionalization has pointed up is that we have been unable to devise a mechanism thus far to allow money to follow patients, wherever they are. For instance, as state hospital populations have diminished and patients have been relocated into community settings, there has been no concomitant shift in funding to allow services to follow the patients. Likewise, while the mentally ill receive Medicaid while in nursing homes, they do not get reimbursed while in state hospitals. In addition, Supplemental Security Income (SSI), for which patients living in apartment programs and single-room occupancy hotels are eligible, is not available in institutional settings. The net result of these inequities is that there has been too little money available in the community for programs to provide care and treatment there, no SSI for persons in hospitals to provide more than the basics, and no monies to upgrade institutional settings. In short, the system seems designed to do exactly what it does—force patients from lousy state hospitals to lousy nursing homes or welfare hotels that have no programs that could prevent the patients from becoming ill again necessitating readmission to the lousy state hospital.

The second problem is that there is not, and never has been, an adequate range of facilities for the mentally ill in the community, each with a range of programs designed for individuals with different problems, levels of functioning, etc. Consequently, patients are placed in what is available (nursing and board-and-care homes) rather than in what they need (halfway houses and communal apartments).

There is not only lack of initial planning in preparation for de-institutionalization, but also a lack of responsibility for and coordination of care for the patient after de-institutionalization. No level of government (city, county, state, federal) assumes responsibility for these patients, and no person or team of mental health workers takes responsibility for coordinating or providing their care—with some worthy and rare exceptions.

In many instances patients are not themselves ready for return to the community. Without a range of stepwise services, we force patients who lack basic skills to survive in our modern communities, to endure countless frustrations and defeats in the process of returning to the community. Unless and until there are adequate habilitation and rehabilitation programs provided inside hospitals preparing patients for the first steps of reentry and adequate community support services outside the hospital to continue the process of growth and return, we are fighting a losing battle where only the lucky survive.

There is a problem of great magnitude in funding services for discharged patients living in the community—indeed for all ambulatory mental patients. The requirements of each governmental agency are different as to which services they will fund for whom. The GAO report[12] goes into detail concerning the programs offered by the major governmental agencies and it is obvious that the regulations and policies applied by each agency force mental health professionals to fit individual patients into set molds rather than provide money for each individual's needs and circumstances. Thus, despite the allocation of millions of federal dollars for the mentally ill to use to meet their various needs—needs such as housing (from HUD), vocational training (Rehabilitation Services Administration) and employment (Department of Labor), supplemental income (SSI) social services (Title XX), and health care (Medicaid and Medicare)—few dollars flow to patients in a sensible, utilizable and unified manner.

Another problem is the continuing strong community resistance to establishing community facilities for the mentally ill. Patients admitted to state hospitals once came from some specific community: but, once hospitalized and institutionalized they are citizens without a neighborhood, and return to their home areas is difficult. In response, mental health providers and patients themselves choose as places of residence ghettos of the de-institutionalized—for examples, the Bowery in New York City, displacing previous populations of alcoholics; decaying communities, as in Long Beach, Long Island, or areas around hospitals, as in towns with such facilities nearby in both New York and California.

The de-institutionalism movement has raised the specter of the collapse of the state hospital system. In response to this threat to thousands of civil service jobs, unions serving largely paraprofessional and nursing staffs have objected strenuously to the move toward community care. At times this has resulted in destructive resistance and unreasoned criticism of community care, but at times the criticism has been logical, constructive, and reasonable in calling for increased job retraining and joint planning for further de-institutionalization.[20]

The de-institutionalization movement has brought into stark relief the seemingly neglected realization that patients who are hospitalized in state facilities are chronic mental patients. They are not simply citizens suffering from a recurrent acute episode of their chronic schizophrenia; they are people who have impaired social functioning, psychological disability, and residual symptomatology. They often have no home, no family, and no friends to whom to return. There is all too often no viable ecological system or social structure awaiting their return. All of the above makes it imperative that we use a model of chronic illness in thinking about this population, and that the goal following resolution of the acute episode must be *care* not cure and *habilitation* before rehabilitation.

SOLUTIONS TO THESE PROBLEMS

It should be apparent by now that there is no simple, single solution to the problems raised by de-institutionalization. Return to the "good old days" of benign, enlightened moral treatment in asylums is unrealistic—time and psychiatry have moved too far. And as Bachrach has pointed out, most critics of the current problems no longer propose simple solutions and "denigrate all alternatives."[5] What is certain is that continuance of "business as usual" will merely worsen the situation for thousands of chronic mental patients.

Solutions must address the problems as they exist, and address each one in turn. Therefore, there must be a range of services available for care of the mentally ill, including some form of protected safe asylum for a small core population as well as a series of graded community facilities and services to permit discharged patients to reach their highest level of functioning *or* to remain for long periods if no progress is attained. A way must be found for monies to follow patients from the hospital to community settings and to be available for actual patients rather than the funds forcing care givers to squeeze patients into agency requirements. There must be a designation of who is responsible for the provision of needed services, ensurance that the services are provided, and coordination of medical and psychiatric care for the de-institutionalized patient. Patients must receive adequate preparation prior to discharge, and the resistance of communities and union members must be addressed. As mental health professionals, we must conceptualize these patients as suffering from chronic illness and/or disability and work to care not cure, convincing our fellow citizens of the merit of this approach.

All of the evidence we have to date indicate that if community programs are to be successful, there must be this joint societal/professional determination to tackle all of the problems outlined and a commitment to bettering patient care rather than merely reforming institutions.[21]

REFERENCES

1. Kramer M: Psychiatric Services and the Changing Institutional Scene. Bethesda, Md, National Institute of Mental Health, 1975
2. Brill H, Patton R: Analysis of population reduction in New York State mental hospitals during the first four years of large-scale therapy with psychotropic drugs. Am J Psychiatry 116:495–500, 1959
3. Meyer NG: Provisional patient movement and administrative data state and county psychiatric inpatient services, July 1, 1974–June 30, 1975. Mental Health Statistical Note No. 132. Rockville, Md, U.S. Department of Health, Education, and Welfare, 1976
4. Cumming J: Screening of admissions. Memo No. 68-27. Albany, New York State Department of Mental Hygiene, 1968
5. Bachrach LL: Deinstitutionalization: An Analytical Review and Sociological Perspective, Rockville, Md U.S. Department of Health, Education, and Welfare, 1976
6. Shapiro JH: Communities of the Alone: Working with Single-Room Occupants in the City. New York, Association Press, 1971
7. Talbott JA (ed): Who will care for the patients? Bulletin of NYSDB's APA 14(5):1–9, 1972; continued in subsequent issues
8. Commission on State-City Relations, The City of New York: State Policy and the Long-Term Mentally Ill: A Shuffle to Despair. New York, the Author, 1972
9. Reich R: Care of the chronically mentally ill: A national disgrace. Am J Psychiatry 130:911–912, 1973
10. The discharged chronic mental patient: A medical issue becomes a political one. Med World News, April 12, 1974, pps. 47–58
11. Schumach M: The New York Times, January-April 1974
12. Returning the Mentally Disabled to the Community: Government Needs to Do More. Washington, DC, U. S. General Accounting Office, 1977
13. The Chronic Mental Patient in the Community. New York, Group for the Advancement of Psychiatry, 1978
14. Glasscote RM, et al: Old Folks at Homes: A Field Study of Nursing and Board-and-Care Homes. Washington, DC, Joint Information Service, 1976
15. Wing JK: Planning and evaluating services for chronically handicapped psychiatric patients in the UK. Paper presented at the Conference on Alternatives to Mental Hospital Treatment, University of Wisconsin, October 1975
16. Lamb HR, Goertzel V: The demise of the state hospital: A premature obituary. Arch Gen Psychiatry 26:489–495, 1972
17. Mesnikoff A: Triangle: A Model for a Public-Private Partnership in a Single System of Mental Health Services in New York City. Unpublished paper.

18. Robbins E, Robbins L: Charge to the community: Some early effects of a state hospital system's change of policy. Am J Psychiatry 131:641–645, 1974
19. Talbott JA: Stopping the revolving door: A study of readmissions to a state hospital. Psychiatry Q 48:159–168, 1974
20. New York Civil Service Employees Association, Task Force on Mental Hygiene: Deinstitutionalization: State and County Policies and CSEA Response. Albany, the Author, 1977
21. Langsley DG, Barter JT, Yarvis RM: Deinstitutionalization—the Sacramento story. Unpublished paper.

PART II

Why State Hospitals Don't Work

5

Beset from Within
and Without

There are literally dozens of limitations placed on persons working in state mental hospitals. As a result, there is less than optimal care for the patients in such institutions. These limitations, or constraints, come from both without and within the institutions. Some arise from the state departments of mental hygiene themselves—which to the external world appear to be internal problems but to the individual facility seem external and "without." The majority of constraints arise not from the institutions themselves, although this is frequently where media attention and therefore cosmetic correction is focused. Rather they are inherent in the existing state bureaucracy or are the result of external pressures. (Figure 5–1 gives a concise and graphic view of the many agencies that influence the worker in a state hospital.) Thus the irony is created whereby an individual hospital's programs can be fashioned to meet the needs of its patient population, but the implementation of them is hampered by external forces. The following sections will discuss some of these contraints.

INTERNAL CONTRAINTS

Staff

The first and foremost constraint on the state mental health facility is its staff. Ancillary health workers, persons who do not hold professional degrees, in general are poorly paid and unappreciated. Mental

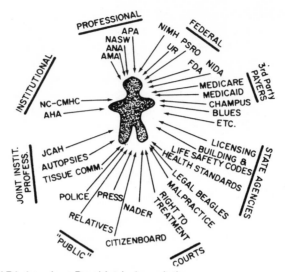

APA-American Psychiatric Association
NASW-National Assoc. of Social Workers
ANA-American Nurses' Association
AMA-American Medical Association
NC-CMHC-National Council of Community Mental Health
    Centers
AHA-American Hospital Association
JCAH-Joint Commission on Accreditation of Hospitals
UR-Utilization Review
NIMH PSRO-Professional Standards
FDA-Food and Drug Administration
NIDA-National Institute of Drug Abuse
CHAMPUS-Civilian Health and Medical Program for Uniformed
    Services
BLUES-Blue Cross and Blue Shield

Fig. 5–1.   Outside forces and the state hospital, (Redrawn with permission from Peele R and Palmer RR: Standards and quality control: Problems and pitfalls. Admin Ment Health 3:148, 1976)

health workers, those who have professional degrees, are, relatively, even more underpaid and unappreciated.

Since the predominant staffing patterns of state facilities have a concentration of nonmedical over medical staff and a greater distribution of nonprofessional or paraprofessional over professional staff, there is an unusually high percentage of the total staff who lack higher educational credentials and often even specialized on-the-job training. This may not be so detrimental in certain rural areas where there may be a more traditional attitude towards community responsibility for deviants and where there may be a higher value placed on the merits of tender, loving care toward society's unfortunates and thus higher caliber workers are found. In metropolitan state facilities this is not usually the case. There one is more likely to find that staff and patient population closely akin in education, ethnicity, socioeconomic background and state of familial and societal disorganization. Although this similarity of background can lead to identification with the patient and familiarity with community resources, it may also lead to the splitting off of the disagreeable parts of one's personality from oneself and the projection of these onto the patients. In this instance there occurs, what is too often seen in such settings, a rejection of patients because they possess the denied traits within oneself (a situation similar to that in prejudice).

In addition, there are cultural and socioeconomic biases against mental illness, leading some mental health workers to regard their patients as malingerers or as persons who lack strong enough wills to overcome their emotions, or as persons who are inherently evil or nasty rather than sick. Since the mental health worker has a low-status job, from the start there is little expectation for intellectual growth and career aspiration. The result is an intrinsically low motivation to learn, change, and act therapeutically. Likewise, because of the lack of either medical/psychiatric education or on-the-job training, most nonprofessionals have few therapeutic tools with which to work, and unless they are unusually motivated, they prefer to concentrate on custodial rather than therapeutic tasks. Here custodial care is being referred to as the rendering of primary need-fulfilling activities, e.g., making sure patients are clean, adequately fed, clothed, housed, and kept warm.

The professional staff, while not usually mirroring the socioeconomic background of the patients, is, nevertheless, different from the dominant professional psychiatric culture. For instance, doctors and nurses are much less likely to be born and educated in the United States than their peers in other mental health settings, and their education and training tends to be less psychiatrically oriented (especially regarding modes of psychotherapy) and more general medically oriented (especially in regards to medication). The other major professionals (psychologists, social workers, and activities therapists) while somewhat closer demographically to their peers in other settings, are usually not in the state system by preference. They are there because of their diminished value in the marketplace. These generalizations, like all such, are subject to individual exceptions, foremost of whom are idealistic and change-oriented mental health professionals who enter the system hoping to alter it for the better.

While many of the differences between professionals working in and out of state mental health sytems hold for the administrative staff

(both medical and nonmedical), there is a significant difference between the two groups. Overall, high-level administrators in state hospitals are better trained for their jobs in a state hospital system, despite
the administrator's tendency to manage mental disorders rather than
oversee active psychotherapeutic treatment. Again, though, many administrators are found in state systems not by preference but because
of other significant reasons: job security, previous training and experience, and value in the marketplace.

Patients

The second major internal constraint is that of the patient population. Few patients are in state mental health facilities because they
prefer them to nonprofit (voluntary) hospitals. As Hollingshead and
Redlich have shown, there is a definite bias toward sending both the
lower socioeconomic patient and the chronic schizophrenic to state
institutions rather than other treatment facilities.[1] As a result, there is a
higher percentage of first admissions, of young patients from higher
socioeconomic classes, and of more acutely ill patients in nonprofit
voluntary or university hospitals than in governmental hospitals. And,
there are more of such patients in county and municipal hospitals and
community mental health centers than in state hospitals. The result of
this trend is that, for the most part, treatment failures from other parts
of the mental health system, find themselves in state hospitals, and
these individuals are older, more chronic, poorer, and with less potential for rehabilitation. As we have shown in Chapter 4, the process of
de-institutionalization has created another level of service or nonser-
vice in community settings, and it is these patients who are frequently
caught in the "revolving door." Not sick enough to warrant perpetual
acute treatment but not intact enough to provide for themselves, they
lead marginal existences in substandard housing. They receive inter-
mittent care from nonprofit, municipal, county, and state hospitals,
with no institution truly providing responsible comprehensive care.

Since the patient population of state hospitals comes from lower
socioeconomic areas (and it is immaterial whether this is due to downward drift[2] or slums creating mental illness)[3] these patients have a
much greater need for medical attention, good nutrition, adequate
clothing, and standard housing. It is precisely these needs that are
often in less than adequate supply in governmental institutions.

Architecture and Location

The architectural setting of state hospitals and the location impose
a constraint on the system. Many existing facilities were built in the

1800s or at the turn of the century, and their massive walls, prisonlike windows and stone floors are unsuited for modern therapeutic activities. It is the rare psychiatric hospital, or any other institution for that matter, whose architecture is flexible enough to change and accomodate to changes in patient needs and treatment resources. But almost anything would be better than the traditional state hospital.

In addition, the site of the hospitals has created problems, whether located far from urban areas or in the midst of a metropolis. The hospitals in bucolic settings are usually too far away from their homes for families to visit easily or for patients to maintain existing familial, social, or vocational ties. Thus, these rural facilities seem increasingly irrelevant, except for patients without social ties who are deemed incurable and unrehabilitable, a label few are willing to place on any patient. Urban state facilities, on the other hand, find their accessibility a major concern. Ease of access has posed problems in terms of violent crimes and drug selling by community residents entering the hospitals.

Role of Superintendent

Another internal constraint is the role of the chief executive in the state facility, the director or superintendent. This role, regardless of the person occupying the position, is a nigh impossible one. Rather than management by results, by differences, by exception, or by any of the other popular managerial techniques, the chief executive in a state facility is forced to practice management by choosing the lesser of several evils, management by crisis, and management by assessment of which constraint to implementing rational programming is most succeptible to manipulation or leverage. The constant pull between internal and external demands unaccompanied by the resources to answer effectively any of the demands leaves its mark. As the author has concluded elsewhere,[4] state hospital directors have short lives of effectiveness, whatever their actual length of tenure in the position. They tend to become cynical, destructively energetic, paternalistic, other-oriented, or absent in interest or fact, or they leave the system altogether.

Programs

The final internal constraint to be considered is program orientation. This refers to the institution's own tendency to be more comfortable and deal more easily with programs that are custodial rather than therapeutic and programs that are directed toward inpatient hospitalization rather than genuine treatment in the community. We have noted that an institution's history is all too often its destiny, and once programs have been set in motion, it is difficult to turn them around. Administrators are all too familiar with the experience of placing new managers in positions where they can change programs, only to have the institutions revert back to their original posture the moment the innovators leave. Institutions, it seems, have memories longer than elephants.

DEPARTMENTAL CONSTRAINTS

Civil Service

The most limiting and frustrating constraint encountered in public hospitals is that of civil service laws and policies. Time after time the administrator is confronted by an inability to hire highly qualified professionals for new or old programs either because of an existing list of candidates for the position, based on competitive examinations for that job title throughout the state, or because the salary is not competitive with the outside world of psychiatry. Time and time again, he or she is confronted with an inability to hire persons with relevant training and interests for innovative programs because of outmoded or inflexible job descriptions. And time and time again, the superintendent and administrative staff are almost totally hampered in firing incompetent and even destructive personnel, because there is nothing "official" written in their personnel records, because they were given adequate performance ratings year after year, because other employees or patients are too frightened to confirm their absences, misbehavior, or incompetence, because the union and/or the employee wants to fight "to the death" any dismissal, and because the process of documenting, counseling, reprimanding, bringing charges, conducting hearings, and following a case through countless appeal levels is more time-consuming, frustrating, and expensive than it seems worth.

There are also built-in disincentives in the civil service system. For example, all hearings must be recorded verbatim, and court stenographers are costly. The union almost without exception backs the employee publicly and with legal assistance while the department of mental hygiene does neither for the hospital administration. Political factors also enter and often override the personnel issues, so that countercharges of racial bias, administrative incompetence, and personal vengeance too often predominate the process. Without question, the intent of civil service laws and regulations is to prevent capricious, biased, or personal factors from entering the hiring and firing process, but the actual end result too often has been to keep ineffective and incompetent staff, to hire the lowest common denominator among applicants, and to place the state hospital, once again at a disadvantage vis-a-vis other mental health services in competing for talented individuals.

Budgeting

Another major crippling departmental constraint is the budgeting process and the overseer budget agency in state executive branches. Because of the incredibly long time between request and allocation of monies, the inflexibility of moving existing monies from one area to another, the inability to exercise discretion and judgment in timing and utilization of funds, and the centralized fiscal control (e.g., the state capitol) rather than local control (in the hospital or even at the program level itself)—because of all these factors there is an inability to implement programs or alter services easily. While hardly unethical and certainly not immoral, administrators "steal" and reallocate money, equipment, and services from one program where they are underutilized to others where they are sorely needed. They bargain with staff members to work long hours for little pay, shorter hours for adequate remuneration, or perform duties outside their stated job descriptions. In a Kafkaesque or Helleresque way it becomes illegal and highly questionable to implement in fact what departmental higher-ups are publicly espousing because the methods of implementation are not available, while it is absolutely safe, and often smart, to do nothing or to resist program change in order to try to provide better patient care (especially in the community) because it reflects the reality of the situation. For example, the installation of concrete walls judged necessary for improved programming of crowded wards seven years ago but which today would hamper activities cannot be stopped because of the time constraints and inflexibility of the budgeting process. Requests for improvements or new programs are not approved solely on programmatic merit or from a zero-base, established on real need; instead they are subject to across-the-board percentage approval or budget cuts. Budgeting maneuvers, such as "rolling over" money or expenses from one year to another, providing money too late in the year to implement programs knowing that budget cuts will surely follow after election day, or denying requests because of minor oversights in paperwork are all too common. Even if monies are obtained, there is still the process of contracting for services or purchasing equipment. It is not the hsopital that is going to use the services or equipment that spends the funds. Rather the central office decides what is best for the local program. Unfortunately, central purchasing offices, throughout the country, seem to have a knack of getting shoddy goods or services— (albeit at low prices)— goods that must later be maintained or replaced and services that must be repeated or accepted reluctantly. The more massive the bureaucracy, the more distant the budgeter from clinician, and the result is waste, not saving, to the taxpayer and a hindrance, not benefit, to the patient.

The Legislature

A constraint that can be classified as neither internal nor external is the state legislature. It too is, in our context, a departmental constraint. While all legislative bodies reflect their constituencies, there is no doubt that they tend to represent their vocal and articulate citizens —whether college-educated, middle-class professionals or welfare mothers—better than they do the mentally ill. It is also unlikely that discharged mental patients will write their representatives praising the state hospitals where they were treated. Rather, legislators receive angry letters from patients, friends, and neighbors about the lack of services or poor care. True, no legislator can be knowledgeable and comprehend all of the issues in depth that he or she is asked to vote on and support. It is ironic, however, that legislators know very little about mental health—one of most important and most heavily funded state programs. Busy legislators, especially those from urban areas, see mental health problems as minuscule in comparison to welfare, education, corrections, housing, day care, etc. In addition, they are carriers of the same prejudices about mental illness that most persons outside the field possess. The fact that commissioners of mental health are appointed by partisan governors makes them vulnerable to the same sort of scrutiny and attack by campaigning legislators that other commissioners and members of the executive are subject to. It is not coincidental that most major exposes in New York State of the State Departmental of Mental Hygiene occur during gubernatorial campaigns.

State Departments of Mental Hygiene

The organizational structure of state departments of mental hygiene presents another barrier to their effective management. Many are top heavy with administrators at the central-office level and understaffed at the hospital level, where operational control should be exercised. At one time in New York State a critic noted that there was one commissioner for each hospital in the state. Because of the demands of the offices and the nature of the persons inclined to accept control-office appointments, few have recent hospital experience and fewer still a continuing daily exposure to treating patients. In fact, recent policies in several states, such as New York, have moved toward precluding the private practice of psychiatry by these professionals, thus effectively ensuring that top administrators will quickly lose sight of patients in their absorption with paperwork and policymaking. The structure is also a barrier because of its inflexibility, with little effort to utilize the top management in task-oriented teams to address certain problems and help individual hospitals at a local level. Thus centralization and distance produce distance and irrelevance of thinking.

Just as the personnel in the state hospital reflect the low status and low marketplace value in which governmental institutional psychiatry is held, the personnel in the central department of mental hygiene reflect the same problems. Often departmental administrators are career civil servants, which is not in itself bad, but which leads to a sameness in thinking and a lack of understanding of (and exposure to) other services and systems. Many administrators are at a disadvantage is understanding the problems encountered in individual institutions because of their lack of familiarity with those institutions over time and their lack of daily clinical experience with patients.

Lack of Stated Goals

Another departmental constraint is the paucity of clearly stated and communicated goals or, if there are goals, an overattention to tangible, quantitative, efficiency-oriented goals and an underemphasis on comprehensive, qualitative, effectiveness-related goals. Consequently, objects, buildings, and figures receive more attention than people, programs, and personal interactions. Emptying hospitals is not a goal that most professionals would articulate, while raising or maintaining the quality of life and level of ability is. Yet we have seen the former phenomenon implemented over the past decade—whether due to the philosophy of community psychiatry (it is better to treat in the home than in the hospital), the impact of legal-judicial decisions (patients must be kept in the least restrictive setting possible), or economic and political factors (transferring the fiscal burden from state-supported hospitals to federally supported nursing homes). De-institutionalization per se, however, has rarely been articulated as a goal by state mental health departments. Unfortunately, what passes as an articulated goal is all too often a superficial platitude with no substantive backing for implementation. For instance, with de-institutionalization, patients are *not* better off in being treated in the community if there is no treatment, no money for treatment, and no housing or social services for them. Or to take another example, the "goal" of individualized treatment plans is a laudable one, but if physicians are so deluged with paperwork, so inadequately trained, and so unsupported by teams of clerical and secretarial workers to assist in the process, there is no individualization, no treatment, and no plan.

No Means to Attain the Goals

The logical next step is establishing the means by which one reaches goals. This is often where the absurdity of the situation is so apparent. Goals can only be attained if there are people, programs, and funding to make them live, otherwise they exist as paper promises. If the goal is improved patient care for persons now residing in the community and one way to reach this goal is a comprehensive network of health, mental health, social and vocational services, it becomes fraudulent to insist on its validity as a means, except as an aspect of administrative fantasy, when there is neither the personnel nor the programs to implement this laudable network or there are no monies or inaccessible monies to do so.

Departmental Regulation

The departmental regulations that supposedly govern the operation of the department's facilities place further constraints on the system. Whereas policies in the private sector are designed to facilitate the handling of problems that one is unfamiliar with, regulations in the public sector are all too often designed to prevent the disasters that incompetent and/or inexperienced persons and institutions may make. Their effect, however, is to lower the level of effective action in all segments of the system. For example, a regulation to require exhaustive review of electroconvulsive treatment procedures, before giving any such treatment, will perhaps stop its indiscriminate use. But it will also increase the paperwork and frustration level of everyone involved, resulting in underutilization of an appropriate treatment modality or, even worse, the utilization of modes of treatment based not on their specificity, usefulness, or applicability, but on their nuisance value or lack of it.

To do nothing becomes a safer course than to do something.

Paperwork

The paper proliferation that engulfs all governmental operations, and that has become an increasing phenomenon in health systems, represents one more departmental constraint. Just as the necessity to feed and clothe patients who are in desperate need diverts the ward worker from therapeutic activities, the necessity to fill out more complex and more numerous forms to certify the need for admission, the need for continuing treatment, the use of treatment modalities, the justification of diagnoses and treatment, etc., allows the frightened professional to concentrate on treating the chart rather than the patient and encourages the diligent professional to routinize the paperwork, e.g., everyone seems to have the same symptoms, diagnosis, and treatment from the written documentation. Again, systems designed to ensure better patient care carry disincentives that bring about in many instances exactly the opposite effect intended. In one hospital the number of pieces of paper necessary for each patient became so numerous that another new form was designed merely to keep track of all of the forms.

Lack of Feedback

A lack of feedback and support from the departmental hierarachy have brought about attitudes of indifference and lack of concern in implementing effective programs. One always hears from the central office if a questionnaire, request, or statistic is late in arriving or if one has made disparaging comments about any aspect of the state government. There is no communication, however, if a conscientious administrator does institute innovative programs, or attempts to change things for the better, or tries to stimulate and encourage personnel in their work. Without backing, or even criticism, one feels as if he or she cannot possibly change the system, so why try. Thus, the message is clearly to keep the paper flowing, keep out of trouble, and cling to the status quo.

Accountability

Concomitant with the lack of feedback from above, is a lack of effective accountability of top management to the higher levels of government. Instead, accountability by harrassment and a fiction of accountability are maintained. For instance, some psychiatrists who are employed by state facilities do not give their fair measure of time or energy to their jobs and some quite legally maintain private practices in the evenings after fulfilling their reponsibilities to the state hospital. Rather than insisting that hospital directors and others hold professionals to their appointed time requirements, it is easier for the bureaucratically inclined to suggest an edict banning all outside practice income. While this will stop the employment of physicians who see private patients, at the tremendous price of losing truly able clinicians, it will leave untouched those who put in their hours apathetically and "cheat" in their delivery of services without practicing privately. True accountability is difficult in a system where not everyone receives appropriate satisfaction from his work and where the tendency is to monitor and police rather than lead and inspire, but until each staff member is held accountable down the line, patients will suffer.

Responsibility Without Authority

A major departmental constraint is the delegation to hospital directors of responsibility without the real authority to carry out the tasks. Too often decisions are made at a central office or regional level that should more appropriately be made locally. For instance, decisions about hospital improvements often are not made by the director of a hospital, in consultation with planners, architects, commissioners, etc., at the regional or central office level. Too frequently they are made by persons in centralized, distant business departments who have little or no idea of the local situation but act on what will pass the legislature or what they think everyone needs this year. Undoubtedly such paternalism is regarded by its possessors as benign, but the result is further diminution of everyone's ability to perform his job.

Responsibility Without Resources

A corollary to responsibility without authority is the assumption of responsibility without the resources to accomplish the task. Here, for example, one is faced by example after example of statements of intent by the department of mental hygiene without adequate backup in terms of money, equipment, and competent personnel to accomplish the stated objective. Medical records must be upgraded, but since there is no money available for medical records librarians, one must either divert a highly paid professional (e.g. social worker) to this work or use an unqualified low-level employee. The resources are lacking to accomplish what is generally agreed to be a worthy task and one for which the director is responsible. On a bigger scale, over the past decade state departments of mental hygiene have carried out a planned program of discharging patients from state hospitals, along with tougher admissions criteria and shorter lengths of stay for patients. This has dramatically reduced hospital populations, but since resources were only sometimes provided—and inadequately at that—to care for these discharged and never-to-be-admitted patients, their plight has become a national scandal.

Accessibility of Decision Makers

An important governmental constraint is the lack of accessibility and visibility of the decision makers. Decisions can be made either by policymakers or by policy implementers and they are frequently made with strangulating success by those in government whose job it is to facilitate the implementation of policy. This is particularly so in regard to decisions affecting mental health services. The legislators and hospital directors who are moderately accessible and visible, do not make many of the crucial decisions. These are made by committees, staffs, accountants, and the invisible gnomes of the budgetary process. Unless these government staffers, bureaucrats and committee persons are as visible and accessible to the public as the legislators who pass the laws and mental health professionals who perform the services, they constitute a huge invisible gap in the decision making process. A gap which the electorate is almost entirely ignorant of. Their accessibility, then, is an important step in pinning down who is responsible for what in the system.

Perpetuating the Department

Just as individual hospitals have a tradition, and changing this is difficult, so do governmental departments of mental hygiene. Their interest is all too often in preserving their jobs and empires, not in providing the best care and treatment possible for those for whom they have a public responsibility. Thus, when program control and funding might better be handled by another agency or level of government (e.g., locally), there is stubborn resistance to relinquishing such control and funding. This, in large part, is the reason why state departments of mental hygiene tend to give over funds to local government, as in California, only on legislative demand.

Politics

Politics affect mental health services and impede their efficient delivery. In our context we do not mean the politics of national or state parties, which most certainly affect mental health but the politics that affect departments of mental hygiene more directly. For instance, it is politically wise for such departments to support cutting costs, even if they are convinced that what is needed for the mentally ill is more money, flexibly utilized. So espousal of trimming expenses is made publicly, with or without actual follow-through in fact. Or, the department states publicly that there is a shocking paucity of this or that program (rehabilitation, rape counseling, etc.), and the department will launch a crusade to combat this problem even though department officials know that adequate funding is not available for such a program. One may condone such behavior from politicians and bureaucrats dealing with highways, energy, and agriculture, but in the human services field it is shameful and cruel. At times it must be openly stated that there are not the resources to combat this or that problem, regardless of its worthiness, and the public and its representatives must decide whether or not to better fund areas based on this knowledge. Promises and false expectations have no place in dealing with human lives.

EXTERNAL CONSTRAINTS

Judicial Decisions

Primary among the external constraints are those imposed by recent judicial decisions. I do not mean to imply disagreement necessarily with the decisions, but rather that their impact is often one of constraining and restricting administrators, albeit often freeing and removing constraints from patients. Decisions such as *Wyatt v. Stickney*, ensuring the right to treatment in state hospitals in Alabama, certainly have a most beneficial intent for all concerned, but translating the need for adequate staffing patterns into real money for staffing is more difficult. Other decisions, such as that which encouraged St. Elizabeth's Hospital in Washington, D.C., to place patients in the least restrictive setting, also are salutary so long as such options truly exist in abundance in the community. However, other decisions, such a *Souder v. Brennan*, which attempted to end peonage in institutions, can result in a troublesome, albeit temporary, discontinuity in hospital programs.

Legal Advocacy Activities

Far ahead of the judicial decisions actually written into law, that place constraints on mental health personnel are the activities of various legal groups that attempt to define and redefine the limits of treatment (involuntary versus voluntary) or modalities of therapy, to set criteria for admission, to fix responsibility to patients, etc. Here the activities of the lawyers involved clearly hamper and harass the administrator, whether intentionally or as a by-product of their primary effort to achieve more rights for patients. Thus, hospital directors often find themselves threatened with legal action, embarrassment, or monetary loss by members of the American Civil Liberties Union or Mental Health Law Project, harassed by staff members of agencies such as New York State's Mental Health Information Service, and badgered by private attorneys—all in the same day. Because of the adversary nature of the law, there is hardly a moment when communication with such persons resembles the psychiatrist's approach of searching for motivation, seeking the widest series of options, and testing and deciding on the most workable alternative. Rather the decision making is along legal models, and the process is time-consuming and wearing.

Governmental Agencies

Another external constraint is posed by governmental agencies, on both a local and federal level. Since funding and licensing the array of services necessary to support the mentally ill is fragmented among so many agencies—with different rules, regulations, criteria for disability, etc.—matching patient needs with appropriate resources is a frustrating experience. Then, too, each agency has its own mission and tends to lose sight of individuals who do not precisely match their ideal target population. Federal, state, and local priorities tend not to be identical, and federal, state, and local procedures are all slightly different. In addition, because they are often merely conduits for funds from the state with no direct control over such monies, local agencies tend to be overzealous in planning, monitoring, and evaluating services. As with all overburdened agencies, they opt for more paperwork and longer meetings rather than intimate contact with populations, service providers, and employees of other governmental agencies.

Accrediting Bodies

Accrediting bodies represent another set of constraints, again often overlapping and sometimes contradictory in content or priority. Along with the many federal agencies that must oversee an institution in order for it to receive funding, there are the Joint Commission on the Accreditation of Hospitals, the various departments and boards of health, and the American Board of of Psychiatry and Neurology whose requirements must be met for a facility to be fully accredited. It is an unusual period of time in which the hospital is not in the state of preparation for an accreditation visit from one or another of these bodies. As with the monitoring and evaluating agencies, the accrediting bodies have their own questionnaires and forms. The time and money spent to deal with these, again, detracts from time and money spent on patients.

State Agencies

Some state constraints that have been classified in the discussion as internal (e.g., civil service) do interfere with the internal functioning of an institution, but the agencies themselves are truly external to the operation. This sort of "control agency" indeed exerts a great deal of control. For instance, New York State's Bureau of Audit and Control, which conducts periodic audits of hospitals, utilizes accounting procedures to evaluate quality factors—a technique long since abandoned by the federal General Accounting Office (GAO), which attempts to wrestle with the problems as they exist rather than compare existing conditions with ideal and perfectionistic expectations. Another alien agency is the state bureau of the budget, which is so far removed from operational problems as to be on another planet. Decisions and priorities decided on by this bureau may well have validity to a hospital's internal structure, but since no direct input is ever sought from line administrators and no feedback returned as to the validity of the rationale behind the decisions, the central bureaucrats might as well be operating without reason. The pervasive influence of the departmental of civil service needs to stressed again. The inapplicability of job descriptions in one area to another, the inflexibility in hiring and firing, and the inflexibility in number of various grades and titles are major barriers to the competent provision of services.

Another state agency that often acts in a manner that complicates and restricts is the office of general services. This office, responsible for purchasing so much of what is necessary to run a state hospital, places constraints in several ways. By contracting with the lowest bidder for craftspeople, it often ensures sloppy or disruptive work. By contracting for the lowest priced equipment, it often finds a bargain in the initial price, but in the long run the cost is greater because of the increasing need for the maintenance of this cheaper equipment. By contracting with the lowest-bidding food vendor it perpetuates the rather mediocre and lifeless foods, beverages, etc., that characterize institutional life.

In sum, state agencies for the most part consistently hamper, not implement, mental health programs. Due to their lack of communications with operational units, their attention to quantification and procedural factors, and their inflexibility and cost consciousness, they manage to further restrict and constrict the responsibility of programs to meet the needs of their patients.

Parents Groups

Parents and relatives groups overtly have the same purpose as that of the mental health administrator—optimal care and treatment of the patient. Under optimal circumstances they can be of invaluable help. Some groups and some relatives, however, are so bent on the negative approach to all issues that they actually hamper, rather than assist the change process. For example, some persons take a stance that hospital or program staff are ipso facto in the wrong, and it is not an explanation but an expurgation that is desired whenever contact is made with the administration. In addition, as is inevitable, those active in such groups frequently use their relationship with key administrators to seek preferential assistance for their relatives. This, of course, results in a VIP syndrome, which is demonstrably bad for patient care.

Hospital Boards

Even one's own board may at times become a constraint. Either through unfamiliarity, distance, or poor communication, the boards of public facilities may respond primarily to media criticism and unwittingly drain staff time and attention in explaining problems and procedures. This interferes with the effective functioning of the hospital or takes away from more important considerations. More often, though, they assist in facilitating program change and help influence community attitudes for the better. Such boards, with their direct link to the governor's office, may also assist in explaining particular needs and programs to that office.

Governor's Office

The governor's office, as a focal point of political pressure, often presents another constraint. The priority of the office is not primarily one of ensuring the availability of adequate human services but of staying successfully in office. Thus, decisions are made, seemingly *ex cathedra*, which have great political import but are antitherapeutic or antiprogrammatic.

Human Rights

All levels of government now have human rights mechanisms, and once again, despite the necessity of such protections based on the history of discrimination over the years, the effect is to provide persons harboring grudges and histories of incompetence another channel through which to counterattack when they are being held accountable and another arena in which to nurse their grievance.

The Press

A major external constraint is posed by the press. A free press, dedicated and balanced, protects the rights of all. Stories about well-run programs, treatment successes, and the complexities of problems posed by ancient institutions grappling with insurmountable problems do not sell newspapers. Scandals, beatings, and little old ladies hallucinating in midtown do. The problem then, is not the press per se, but the members of the press, the pressure for noteworthy news, and the disinterest in the problem patient.

Societal Attitudes

Societal attitudes are another major problem. Most of us are compassionate when it comes to helping someone we know or love who is in trouble, for whatever reason. But mental patients removed and bizarre, represent eyesores to be dealt with by someone else, somewhere else. The public strongly favors that such patients be put away, but this sentiment is not buttressed by the funding necessary to provide adequate care. The move toward de-institutionalization has further alienated the citizenry of this country by its constant reminder that mental patients are an inadequately cared for part of our society.

Fragmentation of Services

The final external constraint is that of the fragmentation of mental health services in most communities. We have federally funded VA hospitals and community mental health centers; state-funded state hospitals, mental retardation units, and aftercare clinics; locally funded municipal or county programs; university and voluntary nonprofit hospitals, funded by a variety of third-party payers; and private hospitals, funded in much the same manner. No state has truly unified the funding, planning, and implementation of mental health services, although most are moving in that direction. As a result, patients shuffle between

the various facilities (the revolving-door syndrome), services lack integration with one another, and no single person or agency has a handle
on the efficiency and effectiveness of mental health services in a particular community. The watchwords of the community mental health
center movement—continuity of care and comprehensiveness of services—remain a hope rather than a reality throughout much of the
country.

REFERENCES

1. Hollingshead AB, Redlich FC: Social Class and Mental Illness: A Community Study. New York John Wiley & Sons, 1958
2. Faris REW, Dunham HW: Mental Disorders in Urban Areas. Chicago,
   University of Chicago Press, 1939
3. Langner TS, Michael ST: Life Stress and Mental Health: The Midtown
   Manhattan Study. New York, Free Press of Glencoe, 1963
4. Talbott JA, Keill SL: A Typology of State Hospital Directors. Unpublished paper.

6
The Politics of
State Hospitals

The problems encountered by state mental hospitals, to a large extent, are created by their role in the political process. Problems such as inadequate funding, changes in mandate, and impractical rules and regulations are directly attributable to the state hospitals' vulnerability to everyday politics.

It would be naive to expect that any governmentally run and supported institution would be allowed to operate free from public scrutiny and control. The political process referred to includes factors outside of expected regulation, scrutiny, and accountability. It includes the intrusion of government into the day-to-day operation of state facilities, the control of program and treatment policies by political appointees lacking familiarity with the health field, and the utilization of the state hospitals' conditions to further candidates' personal political careers during political campaigns.

I must make it clear that I am not advocating unbridled freedom from accountability—in fact, I favor the opposite. I maintain that 100 years of political accountability has compounded, not remedied, the problems faced by state hospitals and that some other form of public accountability must be devised if we are to end the cycle of underfunding, overregulation, misdirection, and scandalous revelation of the inadequacies of state mental facilities.

POLITICS AND MENTAL HEALTH PROFESSIONALS

Mental health professionals, particularly psychiatrists, are untrained and frequently ill equipped to become involved with and educate legislators, governmental aides, and legislative committee staffs as to the problems regarding the treatment of mental illness and their potential solutions. Most psychiatrists are comfortable in one-to-one situations, are competent to treat or direct treatment of the mentally ill, and talk easily and enthusiastically with peer professionals about their work. They frequently become tongue-tied, defensive, and heated, however, when answering the most elementary questions asked by persons outside the field. When such questions are posed in a quasi-adversary manner, as during budget hearings, investigations, committee meetings, or confirmation proceedings, the problems are frequently aggravated rather than clarified and solved.

In addition, most health professionals start from a conceptual and informational scientific base that assumes that medicine is trying to cure illness utilizing the best available therapeutic tools. Questions concerning those tools or their scientific certainty are thus met with impatience and/or contempt, colored by anger and defensiveness. Medical educators, used to the hardest questions imaginable when posed by first-year medical students, lose their ability to explain, justify, and educate the questioner who may be a 40-year-old lawyer or legislative aide.

Mental health professionals, as a result, frequently become involved in dialogues with legislators that are extremely unproductive for both. Since legislators, at this point in time, are the representatives of public responsibility, more time has to be spent with legislators and their aides by persons comfortable with this educational-informational approach in a nondefensive way.

THE POLITICS OF LEGISLATORS

Legislators are political animals, and were they otherwise they would be back in their law offices or private enterprises in short time. Their role is, therefore, split— as politicians they must get elected and stay in office, while as legislators they must represent their constituents as best they can. These two roles are often congruent when it comes to the field of mental health. In campaigning one needs issues to highlight the necessity for one's election—and the deplorable state of most state mental institutions is an ever available target. It is, therefore, natural for every new political candidate to hold a tour and news conference at a local state hospital and promise the electorate that things will change once he or she gets into office. The role of legislator, however, ensures that this will not happen. While mental health constitutes the largest single portion of the state tax dollar in many states, by no means does the legislature apportion a similar amount of time and effort to its expenditure. This is due to several reasons: the press of new legislation to solve emergent problems, the sheer magnitude of the number of concerns facing the legislature, and, most importantly, the lack of a strong constituency pressing legislators to act on the behalf of mental patients.

Mental patients do not write letters to their state representatives or to newspapers; they do not picket or demonstrate in front of state capitols; and they have no lobbying or public affairs representatives. As opposed to labor, businesses, and the professions—which have all these methods at their immediate disposal—they are almost completely powerless to affect the political process. Even compared to other have-not groups—alcoholics, prisoners, or welfare mothers—they have no clout. The mentally retarded, so long neglected in America, at last have benefited from effective political efforts, due to the impact their mentally intact parents have had on a sympathetic public. The mentally ill do not have such a body of mentally intact relatives, due to the complex socioenvironmental and genetic etiology of serious mental illness. In addition, there is much less public sympathy for the mentally ill. As a result, they constitute one of the truly powerless constituencies in our society. When persons working in state facilities lobby for their hospitalized charges, their efforts are seen as self-serving. Even professional societies are suspect because of their supposed vested interest in economic and status issues rather than patient care.

THE GOVERNOR'S OFFICE

The thrust behind an interest in the state hospital system may come either from the legislative or the executive branch of government. While most governors seek out a competent commissioner for mental health and encourage this individual to chart the course of mental health services, there are times that the governor's office itself takes charge. The reasoning is understandable; the frustration at having to deal with a large encrusted bureaucracy leads to the fantasy that someone at a higher level can cut through all the red tape and "really change things." Serious and chronic mental illness, however, represents a complex area, not readily understood by reading a few books, sitting in on a few hearings, or by possessing good intentions. The history and functioning of the state mental hospital system is equally difficult to grasp without extensive experience and day-to-day exposure. Therefore, initiatives emanating from the governor's chambers, while often aided by informed professionals, tend to offer legal (e.g., lawyers controlling admissions procedures rather than physicians) or administrative (e.g., the consolidation, decentralization, or introduction of new managerial techniques or personnel) solutions rather than clinical or programmatic ones. As such, they usually make the situation worse since the essential problems remain untouched.

CITY/STATE POLITICS

Mental health services are sometimes caught in the battle between state and local authorities over planning, implementing, and monitoring services. Nowhere is this more evident than in New York City. For at least 10 years the city and state governments have been involved in various battles over jurisdiction, control, and adequacy of services. This battle has raged regardless of which party is in power in either place and has involved welfare, Medicaid, and the administration of New York City's government itself.

De-institutionalization and dumping of patients are the issues over which mental health services have become most involved in the fight. It is apparent in retrospect that state hospitals discharged patients to New York City neighborhoods without there being either state or local services in adequate number or range to provide appropriate community care. As a result, the emergency services of the local (municipal and voluntary) hospitals began to reflect the discharged patient population rather than their previous diverse acute-onset group. Even after de-institutionalization decreased the hospital rolls, the money theoretically saved by the need for fewer staff and building less space was not passed on to the localities. The local hospitals then became "chronicized." They fought back by trying to send patients to state facilities as quickly as possible rather than treat them for adequate periods of time with appropriate methods, as they had in the past. As one critic observed, the only difference between the state and city hospitals was that the state provided chronic custodial care and the city acute custodial care. Most recently the state and city mental health authorities decided that it was the voluntary hospitals who were not doing their share, and they moved in 1977 to slow down direct admissions from voluntary hospital emergency rooms to both state and city hospitals. This will result in "chronicized" voluntary hospitals. One can safely predict that this will lead to the development of a new entity—emergency custodial care. All of this might be somewhat amusing if buck-passing occured in other government areas, but with mental health services it will only result in patients being hurt.

Another battleground involves who should plan mental health services. During the early 1970s, the important task, if one listened to city and state mental health agencies, was that of program planning. No one, it seemed, wanted to provide services, but everyone wanted to plan or coordinate them. A new industry was created—that of planning. While the persons occupied in this endeavor carried different names—the state called them program analysts and the city, senior consultants (there seemed to be no junior ones)—they did precisely the same thing. The situation reached the height of absurdity when at one catchment area meeting there were more "planners" than service providers. To the observer it seemed obvious that the task of providing services had become too onerous for the governmental agencies and the retreat to fighting over who planned was an effective defense against grappling with their failure to provide services.

SOME OBSERVATIONS ABOUT THE BASIC DILEMMAS

There are two basic dilemmas regarding politics and the state hospital. First, state hospitals have a public health role and are expected to care for all regardless of need, *but* they do not have the resources to fulfill their responsibility nor the political means to obtain those resources. Second, the patients who are consumers of these services have no way of influencing the provision of their own services. Thus, the two populations in the system—the care providers and the care recipients—have little or no power to suggest, influence, or provide what is needed. If any business were to abide by these rules, it would soon be bankrupt.

What then can be done? First, the hallowed administrative dictum that no one can be responsible for a task if not given the authority and resources to accomplish it should be invoked. State hospitals should not be faulted for providing inadequate services; the legislators and governmental agencies that limit their authority and resources should. Second, a process of effective consumer advocacy must be developed that can perform the same functions that labor or business lobbyists do

—advocate for adequate mental health services, educate the public and the legislators, and lobby for appropriate and adequate care and treatment. Parents and relative groups have begun this task in some areas but, as noted previously, are impotent in contrast to other groups who lobby the legislature. The parents groups have concentrated on the providers of services (directors, commissioners, etc.) rather than work on the more difficult but logical target for activity—society and its elected representatives. Lastly, a process must be found for an accountability procedure that ensures that the public gets its value for each tax dollar spent on mental hospitals, a process which would not be vulnerable to abuse by headline-hunting auditors or campaigning politicians.

Continuing the charade of expecting state facilities to take care of the seriously and chronically mentally ill without adequate resources and then scapegoating them for their failures to do so is clearly neither in the public's nor the patient's interest.

What is needed is an ongoing procedure whereby goals are defined, services monitored, feedback provided, and reappraisal of goals made in such a manner that it becomes clear what taxpayers are getting for their dollar and how much more would be needed to provide optimal services and care.

But this is not an easy task and will not happen without the public's insistence on improvement.

7
Mentalities

There are a number of mental attitudes, or "mentalities," that predicate much of the activity undertaken by governmental psychiatric facilities. None of the mental attitudes or sets discussed in this chapter is unique to the mental health system, but their prevalence is an important factor in the operation of the system.

Attitudes, values, expectations, and perceptions are all important in the way each member of a mental health center views his or her job, the facility's responsibility, and the goals of the organization as a whole. A simple example concerns the way people refer to each other in different settings. At a prestigious graduate school in the medical sciences people refer to almost all others in the system as colleagues, indicating respect, common orientation and training, and willingness to work with and understand others' work. In the state hospital system, however, co-workers are called employees, indicating their primary role as hired hands, their being replacable and interchangeable, and their distance from the speaker.

The mentalities to be discussed constitute mental attitudes underlying the observed behavior in state mental hospitals. Each has a direct effect on behavior, and each interacts with the other mentalities to produce cumulative effects.

THE FACTORY MENTALITY

The most striking mentality in state hospitals is that of the "factory" mentality, that is, the attitude that what one does is not a professional task but a common job. As a result, state hospital workers regard their positions in a mechanical and detached way. Absences and lateness are viewed as having little or no effect on hospital operations. The fact that patient care is affected seems not to matter. Work is calculated in terms of the number of hours in a day rather than the amount of work necessary to accomplish a task or help a patient. Lest some readers assume that I am talking primarily about the attitudes of nonprofessionals or paraprofessionals, let me emphasize that persons at all levels and with all sorts of training fall prey to this attitude. It is startling to hear psychiatrists applying for jobs ask first about sick days, fringe benefits, and pensions and last about patients, treatment modalities, and service programs.

Since the underlying attitude is that a state hospital job is like that in a factory, the hospital staff person logically becomes an "employee," puts in hours, and tries to retain his or her job, causing as few changes as possible. For the private practitioner, every new patient and additional patient hour constitute another challenge and additional income, and most private practitioners work a fairly heavy schedule. For the state hospital doctor, however, the opposite prevails; the state doctor often tries to see as few patients as possible and to live as relaxed a life as possible.

Since there is little or no concern for patient improvement or pride in one's work, there is little incentive to work hard. The profit motive is absent, and no method of profit sharing can be devised to improve productivity even if one accepts the mentality. As a matter of fact, productivity might lead to abolishing jobs. The harder the staff in state hospitals work to improve the care of patients, the greater the staff worries that without a high census in the hospital their jobs will vanish. So the net result is a subtle but definite message—keep the beds full, the patients ill, and the schedule uncomplicated and unhurried.

THE BUREAUCRATIC MENTALITY

Bureaucratic thinking pervades the mental health system. This mentality forces an attention to organizational detail, policy, procedure, and structure at the expense of individuals, flexibility, and utilization of the unique assets of human energies. The reverence for form

over content, for structure over function, and for statistics over mean-
ing has telling effects on the mental health system.

At higher levels what is important is the bureaucracy and organization qua organization—not the goals of the organization, not the
people it is or was intended to serve, and not the provision of services.
The ultimate expression of the bureaucratic mentality is a devotion to
perpetuating the bureaucracy at the expense of all else. Thus it becomes more important to submit budgets that will be accepted than
budgets that reflect true needs; it is more important to report high
numbers of people processed through the system than demonstrate
high quality of care; and it is more important to prevent the disaster
rather than foster growth and change.

At lower levels the bureaucratic mentality finds firm rooting by
demonstrating the necessity of following the book, whether the reference to clinical care or administrative procedure, and is exemplified
by an attention to paperwork and record keeping at the expense of
seeing and treating patients and by the clinging to job descriptions and
job limitations as methods of avoiding dealing with patient and program needs. Clinicians are extremely resentful of the business administration aspects of the bureaucracy (e.g., requisitions, personnel forms,
statistical reports, etc.), but they too subscribe to and apply the bureaucratic mentality. There are ample examples of its impact among
them—e.g., attention to psychopharmacological details, inflexible and
standardized treatment plans, and the emphasis on treating the chart
rather than the patient.

THE POLICE MENTALITY

There is a great and natural temptation when things do not seem to
be working right in large systems to stop attending to individuals and
programs that attempt to achieve certain goals and to begin to monitor,
check, police, and scrutinize as much as possible. This is not program
evaluation in the usual sense, whose purpose is to improve the quality
of patient care. It is system policing, whose purpose is a further attempt to control and monitor a system that seems out of control and
incapable of management.

For example, the usual approach (outside state hospitals) to the
problem of a physician's seemingly flagging interest in his duties is to
talk it over and try to understand the problem. A typical response in a
state facility would be to begin to document any pecadilloes or overt
signs of the problem, write up such observations, and attempt to moni-

tor or police the person's activities. Thus, all too often in giant-sized institutions, administrators find themselves not seeing patients, not leading staff discussions, not initiating new programs, or not participating in case conferences or other teaching activities. Instead they are involved in supervising subordinates who are presumed not to be doing their jobs, in monitoring statistics, discharge rates, and absences, in checking parking lots early in the morning and late in the afternoon, and in dropping by wards unexpectedly on weekends and at night not to meet the staff or see the patients at off-peak hours, but to check up on and police the system. Policing replaces caring, monitoring replaces evaluating, and personnel surveillance replaces treatment supervision.

THE SURVIVAL MENTALITY

The determination to survive is a powerful theme in many who work in the system. Survival in the face of adversity is obviously a very valuable human trait, but when it becomes the primary goal in professional life, it stifles creativity, growth, and risk taking.

Persons who feel a strong sense of their need to survive the adversity in the state system tend to make as few waves as possible in the hopes of surviving for as long as possible; they act conservatively and cautiously so as not to draw others' attention; and they stick as closely as possible to policy guidelines and traditional procedures in order to outlast and outlive new movements. Since one can avoid error only by inaction, this is all too frequently the course followed.

THE PROPERTY MENTALITY

Many in government service possess a property mentality—that is, a respect for property, buildings, and structures exceeding that for programs, people, and services. This need not be an either/or situation, but the evidence is clear that, more often than not, more attention is paid and more funding is supplied to structures than to programs. A glaring example is that of a state children's hospital built at great cost to the taxpayers but insufficient funding to permit hiring the staff to carry out the programs. Another common occurence is the purchase of expensive medical equipment without commensurate funds for skilled staff to operate and maintain such equipment. Still another is attention to fire extinguishers and safety chutes and disregard for patient amenities such as modern shower stalls, toilet seats, and private clothes storage space.

THE QUANTIFICATION MENTALITY

Persons who demonstrate the quantification mentality look for efficiency indices (input/output) rather than effectiveness (input/impact) and tangible, demonstrable, hard facts rather than subjective, intuitive, softer data. Attention is paid to quantity not quality, to numbers not substance, and to appearance rather than inner workings.

Thus, to many it is more important how many patients are seen by an outpatient clinic, how many admissions and discharges there are in a period of time, and what the length of stay is than how well patients are being treated, how much recovery is shown, and how high a quality of treatment and care is offered. Counting the number of minutes spent between patient and therapist is certainly easy to do, but determining the quality of the interaction and degree of improvement shown is much more difficult. The tendency in most state systems is to hope that quantity is better than nothing, to pursue the collection of data, and to maintain that it is the number of bodies working and amount of dollars spent that will result in good patient care. In this manner issues of competence, of inadequately trained and motivated staff, and of flexibility in hiring staff need not be faced.

THE NIHILISTIC MENTALITY

The nihilistic mentality holds that to do nothing is better than to do something because almost any action will result in negative results. This is a highly adaptive mentality, which results in stagnation of the system, and is a self-fulfilling prophesy because to "goof off" is justifiable, smart, and adaptive.

For example, if there is a crisis, if one does nothing, the crisis may pass, someone else may deal with it, or it may find expression elsewhere. In any case, one's own ability to handle it never comes into question. Keeping a low profile and letting someone take care of a problem is rewarded by continuing service, whereas evidence of human difficulty dealing with problems may lead to one's own and other's realization of the difficulty and, therefore, one's vulnerability.

8
Structural, Procedural, and Operational Obstacles

In the previous three chapters, the major reasons for the difficulties that state mental hospitals have in fulfilling their responsibilities have been discussed. These were arbitrarily grouped into constraints, political factors, and prevailing mentalities. In this chapter, another group of obstacles that state institutions invariably encounter will be addressed. The governmental and bureaucratic structures in which state hospitals are located themselves impede the functioning of the institutions. Some of the obstacles imposed are related to the organizational structure inherent in either the state government or mental health departments and some to the tradition, operation, and functioning of these structures. Students of administrative theory will recognize that issues such as authority, responsibility, and accountability are intimately related to the organization's structure, while budgeting, priorities, and attitudes are more related to procedural and operational factors.

THE AUTHORITY/RESPONSIBILITY/
ACCOUNTABILITY PROBLEM

Inherent in the position of state hospital superintendent or director is the inbalance of the executive's authority, responsibility, and accountability. While many critics of the state mental hospital system point out that the traditional state facility is managed in an authoritar-

ian manner, with centralization of decision making and lack of open
communication, in point of fact, most directors do not have the authority to do much else but manage their day-to-day operations. Allocating
money, formulating policy, and relating to others in the mental health
system—all of which are necessary elements to control if the hospital
is to change—are outside a director's purview. Instead, only circumscribed programmatic and clinical areas are within his domain. In addition, the director's hands are so tied by constricting and seemingly
arbitrary laws, rules, and regulations that to fire incompetent staff, to
move monies into new and needed programs, and to shift resources to
meet changing need becomes so difficult that it is much easier to stick
to the status quo.

As for responsibility, here again there is a paradox. The public
health responsibility vested in directors mandates their responsibility
for large numbers of chronically and severely mentally ill, but they are
usually not given the tools or resources commensurate with the magnitude of the task, again assuring the failure of the hospital to attain its
obvious goals. So many tools are not available (e.g., the power to hire
and fire to insure high-quality staff) and so many resources lacking (e.g.
community alternatives to in-hospital treatment) that the responsibility
implicit in the job is ludicrously out of balance with the ability to carry
out that responsibility. The common response to such an imbalance is
to cut one's losses, attempt stability and survival as primary goals, and
pray that one's responsibility is never questioned by the public.

Such public accountability is irrational in mental health. Despite
the interest of the press in the inadequacies and horrors found in state
hospitals, the public usually is unwilling to back the changes necessary
to alter those conditions. Thus, there is occasional accountability to
the press and accreditating bodies, but full accountability cannot be
forthcoming since there is no attempt by either the legislative or executive branches to provide the resources and procedures to enable state
hospitals to fulfill their public responsibility and to hold the elements in
the system accountable. Accountability is only possible when it is (1)
accompanied by adequate resources and (2) consistantly expected up
and down the chain of command.

The most glaring lack of public accountability is that of the legislators, who vote the funds, laws, and policies that control the activities
of departments of mental hygiene. Accountability is almost equally
absent in the relationship between mental health departments and their
state hospital directors and that between the directors and their staffs.
Everyone below the level of the legislature plays a game—aware that
they are sitting on a powder keg but unwilling to risk loss of job and
reputation by baring the facts.

In administering state facilities only rarely does anyone utilize what is generally accepted as sound administrative procedure: the zero-based budget and program.   Instead the practice is to base operations on what is imposed from "above"—existing budgets, civil service laws, and departmental policies. If the needs of the patients served as the base and then the resources and tools necessary to provide quality care and treatment were calculated, responsibility and accountability for care and programs might at least stand a chance of being addressed. With such an approach, if resources were not allocated, then accountability would be more circumscribed and responsibility defined as much more limited. But a start would have been made at facing the reality of the situation. Now, since everyone below the level of the legislature knows that the resources and tools are inadequate, no one really holds subordinates accountable, expects them to be responsible for the care of their patients, or emphasizes their limited authority.

BUDGETARY OBSTACLES

The budgets of departments of mental hygiene are often skewed in such a way as to reward the wrong things. For instance, for years bed occupancy, rather than quality of care or evaluation of the job done, was the basis for funding. Until recently, no mental health facility was evaluated in terms of patient outcome. This will be feasible soon. Then, perhaps, funding can have a productive basis. Certainly de-institutionalization has demonstrated the inability of an entire system to provide quality care, and quality rather than quantity must be discussed.

Another example of the wrong emphasis in budgeting is the tendency to relate budgets to the number of inpatient beds. As a result, state facilities are rewarded for their inpatient activity rather than their ability to care for people in whatever setting is most appropriate. Budgets should be related to the needs of the population at risk, to their needs relative to the services available, and to the number of patients treated on an ambulatory basis, and the amounts arrived at figured on a cost-reimbursement basis as is done in the private hospital sector.

Another faulty reward system involves efficiency and inefficiency. Since numbers are easier to understand than program descriptions, funding is more often based on numbers of admissions or discharges, lengths of stay, and number of visits than on the quality indices of recovery rates, levels of functioning, ability to follow-up patients, provision of aftercare services, etc. Seemingly "efficient" facilities that run large numbers of patients through their "assembly-line" programs are rewarded more than those that spend more time with fewer patients and may obtain better clinical outcomes.

If monetary reward-punishment systems were enforced with facilities that performed well or badly, the persons who would suffer from decreases in funding would be the patients—not the ineffective staff. Therefore, government administrators are reluctant to cut funds to an ineffective hospital, feeling correctly that this would only aggravate the situation. The solution to this might be to relate the income of the administrators to productivity, to replace ineffective leadership, or to provide outside assistance or control.

THE WRONG PRIORITIES

The degree to which priorities are skewed in state hospital systems can scarcely be appreciated by the outsider. One would expect that given the level of disability, socioeconomic deprivation, and extent of chronicity and severity of mental illness afflicting the state hospital population, the ultimate priority would be quality treatment and patient care, innovative and forceful clinical activities, and energetic problem solving and treatment planning. Nothing could be further from the truth. Instead, the focus is frequently on maintaining the status quo, on individual survival, on professional territoriality, and on the avoidance of trouble.

This skewing of priorities is reflected in the larger system as well. Almost never are communications from higher-ups addressed to clinical care issues, and there is never an articulated concern for attaining the highest quality of care. Attention is paid, instead, to food and sanitation, to policies and procedures, and to reporting of all sorts of statistics from detailed demographic data on the patients to the racial composition of the staff. As a result, the attitude engendered is similar to that during the Viet Nam war when body counts were inflated or invented and statistics replaced thinking.

In addition, the resources of state departments of mental health are frequently perverted to narrow ends. For instance, education and training funds are more often used to hire cheap labor from developing nations (labor that rarely returns to the countries that need it) rather than educate young American psychiatrists to care for the chronically and severely mentally ill. Public information and public affairs' efforts are more often used to justify a department's shaky policies (e.g. inadequate security forces, de-institutionalization, or lack of effective treatment) than to alter public opinion about the mentally ill or to inform the populace about the difficulties in treating the severely ill.

Two of the reasons for the priorities being so skewed are the difficulty encountered in treating this population of impaired patients and the frustration involved in dealing with its members. Physicians, faced with overwhelming tasks, withdraw to administrative offices; clinicians, frustrated by the lack of resources, take to gathering statistics and treating the chart; and attendants, untrained and ill equipped to cope with severe mental illness, retreat to polishing floors, controlling behavior, or drinking coffee. The advent of effective antipsychotic medication has eliminated bizarre behavior and florid symptomatology, but it has not altered the patients' basic impairment in functioning once back in the community or the need for the treatment staff to maintain contact to insure that treatment and rehabilitation will continue. Follow-up, continued support, and energetic community efforts cannot be prescribed like medication; they must be an inherent responsibility of the treatment staff.

THE IRRATIONALITY OF THE SYSTEM

The mental health system (or nonsystem, especially when it comes to the state mental health component of that system) has never been noted for its rational approach to problem solving. That the system operates at all may be a tribute to the better nature of humans, given the system's dependence on politically determined policies and budgets, its tasks, which are conflicting and unrealistic, and the fact that it is so poorly understood by the public, elected officials, and even its peer professionals.

To the observer, the system seems to act counter to its own best interests and often in an irrational manner. Rewarding facilities that do not provide quality care, punishing patients whose illness prevents them from cooperating with treatment efforts, and promoting clinicians to administrative positions once they have proven their effectiveness in treating this population, all seem to be counterproductive.

In addition, developments occur in the system that seem unrelated to perceived needs. Budgets, for example, are not cut because the job has lessened and money is no longer needed, but because there is an economic crunch. Statistics are suddenly requested not because clinicians need them to provide better patient care, but because statisticians speculate that they might reveal some trends. Or directors are told their population will go down in the next five years not because data has demonstrated a change in their service area's needs, but because some functionary senses a statewide or nationwide trend, which everyone must participate in. Cause is disconnected to effect, and the actions taken seem irrational in respect to the true situation.

PREVAILING ATTITUDES

There are several prevalent attitudes that have such tenacity and persistance that one must assume they are inherent in the state mental hospital system. Most prominent of these are the opinion that high officials in the department of mental health never do what they say they will and, more revealing, the opinion that no one cares that if they do or do not. For example, the moment state or regional officials announce a new program or effort (rape counseling centers, facilities for violent patients, or alcoholism or drug abuse services, etc.), veteran observers shake their heads cynically and proclaim that there will not be enough expertise, resources, or funding to implement the program fully, and if the program fails, neither the administrators nor their superiors will care. In short, they imply that there is no shame among these public servants.

Throughout most state systems there is an attitude of overwhelming pessimism that the job cannot be done. Such a stance inevitably leads to the rationalization that, therefore, one need not even try. Too often the prophecy becomes self-fulfilling and destroys whatever chance for change exists. Examples of this are the attempts to reduce inpatient beds by utilizing alternatives to inpatient hospitalization, such as day or night hospitals. Before these facilities are adequately funded or staffed, a decision is reached that the job cannot be done.

The most discouraging attitude, however, is that nothing in state hospitals is really worth doing anyway, it all will come to naught. While most officials in state departments will publically deny this attitude, they betray their adherence to it by their actions. For example, rather than fight to be able to hire a director of quality by increasing the salary level, obtaining a medical school liaison, or promising extra assistance in terms of outside consultants, extra staff, or new program monies, they too often settle for the best person who applies for the job. The author cannot conceive of a profit-making business or nonprofit academic department in a university settling for the best of a bad bunch; rather they define the sort of person they think is best for the job, and set out to find that person, regardless of obstacles.

LOW STATUS

Previous sections have considered the low status that state hospitals, state hospital jobs, and state hospitals activities are accorded by society as well as professional groups. In the present discussion low status refers specifically to (1) the low priority that state legislators place on the state hospital system in their list of concerns (in large part because this wheel does not squeak) except in election years, (2) the low priority that state departments of mental health place on patient care, in large part because they feel ill equipped to treat the severely and chronically mentally ill, and (3) the low standing such governmental agencies as budget or civil service place on quality and outcome, in large part because they are remote from the realities of how difficult and stubborn are the problems of care and treatment of the state hospital population.

Because mental health has such a large uncontrolled chunk of the state budget, because its problems are so poorly articulated and understood, and because it has no citizen lobby of note, its low status within the bureaucracy is perpetuated by continuing administrative constraints, budgetary cuts, and thoughtless policies.

This part has attempted to isolate and discuss the individual issues and problems faced by state mental hospitals in terms of the constraints, politics, mentalities, and structural obstacles that affect them. In the next part we will address the process of change in the state system and what changes may be possible or realistic, given the present state of affairs.

PART III

What Can Make
Them Work

9

The Struggle for Change
in State Hospitals

The struggle to change state hospitals for the better is challenging as well as exhausting. Although the descriptive literature regarding how to change institutions has proliferated over the years, little has had direct application to the state hospital situation. This chapter will consider why state hospitals are different, the types of change that affect state facilities, the prerequisites for change, the fate of change agents, and the resistances to change. It will end with a basic bibliography for the change-minded. A caveat for the reader, while the word *change* is frequently used without its modifier—for the better—in all instances improvements in the situation are meant, not change that is retrogressive or lateral.

STATE HOSPITALS ARE DIFFERENT

State hospitals combine the features of a public agency with those of a mental health service; therefore they sum the constraints applicable to both types of organizations.

Golembiewski has pointed out that change in public agencies is hampered by several constraints: the need for security and secrecy, the reliance on procedural regulations and caution, a legal orientation to administration (e.g., civil service rules), the weak linkage between political appointments and career employees, the multiple access to decision makers, and the dependence of the system on professional managers.[1] Feldman has noted the factors that make administration in mental health different from that in other areas: mental patients carry an enormous stigma, the boundaries of the field are more difficult to define, the product is intangible and consists primarily of hope and confidence, a highly dependent population is the focus, there is a unique patient/therapist relationship in addition to other relationships, and the professions involved deal with difficult problems using difficult personnel.[2]

In summing these obstacles to change for a state hospital, one arrives at more than simple addition would lead one to believe. In addition to the governmental constraints (e.g., civil service, regulations, and politics) and the mental health features (e.g., intangible product, difficult problems, and a stigmatized population), several other factors discourage change in a state hospital. These have been amply described in Chapters 5 and 8. The most pertinent to the present discussion are the hospitals' antiquated structures (administrative and architectural), their public health responsibility, their population of chronic mental patients, and the lack of responsiveness by both society and medicine to the most severely and chronically mentally ill. As Fowlkes has pointed out, society's creation and maintance of custodial mental hospitals is dependent on powerful forces, forces that do not individually or collectively lend themselves to easy alteration.[3] This factor is one reason why, while internal and external changes may affect them it is probably not until there are systems or societal changes that the total functioning of the state hospitals can be improved.

TYPES OF CHANGES IN STATE HOSPITALS

There are four types of changes that affect state facilities: internal, external, system, and societal.

Internal Changes

Internal changes are those within the purview of the individual hospital director and/or the hospital staff. They include initiating and modifying programs, upgrading staff, and implementing new hospital procedures and policies. Even a supposedly minor change may have a large impact. One administrator changed the practice of the hospital director signing all correspondence leaving the hospital and insisted that individuals sign their own letters, requests, and replies. The previous practice had been justified by the concern that improper information might be conveyed to the wrong persons, that mistakes in clinical judgment or grammar might be revealed, and that monitoring was needed. The rationale really concealed another motivation—that of control of all official communication between the institution and the rest of the world. The cessation of this centralized function conveyed a powerful message to the staff, despite its seeming triviality.

External Changes

Only a thin line separates internal and external changes. For instance, in one state hospital the director proposed changing from a geographically unitized system to functional units (e.g., by age, diagnosis, and level of functioning) to permit staff to concentrate on definable rehabilitation objectives and unify inpatient and outpatient programs. He assumed that this was an internal change. While it did not necessitate external (departmental) approval, it did depend on it for successful implementation. He was informed that such a change was not only *not* within his authority, but was contrary to one of the basic tenets of the department: geographic unitization.

External changes, then, are those that the hospital itself does not control but, rather, are within the scope of the higher (departmental) authority. Such changes usually involve departmentwide procedures or policies with which individual facilities may or may not agree but to which they are bound. An example of a policy that departmental officials initiated but that had little institutional, and no extra-system, support was the policy initiated in 1968 in New York State to stop admitting persons over 65 to state hospitals who did not have acute psychiatric illnesses felt to be responsive to acute psychiatric intervention. Other examples of external changes include uniform reporting and monitoring of untoward incidents (e.g., injuries, death, etc.), regulation of therapeutic modalities (e.g., electroconvulsive therapy or multiple drug use), and new policies in regard to working hours, career ladders, or fringe benefits.

An examination of the examples given of internal and external changes reveals that all of the internal changes involved loosening or decentralizing maneuvers, whereas the external innovations cited involved tightening or constricting ones. Lawrence and Lorsch have pointed out that in recent years in the field of organizational theory there have been about an equal number of innovations that could be classified as either loosening or tightening operations.[4] In state mental hospitals, however, it seems that most loosening (and by inference, creativity) has occured at the institutional level, while most tightening (and thus constriction) has come from above and without.

System Changes

Changes involving the entire mental health system, on a state or national level, private or public, are system changes. The attempt to alter the funding formula for counties in New York State so that the counties would become the central provider of services, placing state facilities in a role of quasi-hotel operators, was such a change. National changes of this nature usually include more widespread funding initiatives—such as that by Medicaid in reimbursing with federal funds those mental patients sent to nursing homes, thus expediting the deinstitutionalization process. It would be a system change if national health insurance covered medical services for mental patients wherever they resided. This reimbursement arrangement would have a profound effect on state hospitals, whose patients would probably prefer to be treated elsewhere.

Societal Changes

Societal changes are less prevalent but more profound than the previous three categories. Current attitudes about the severely and chronically mentally ill, ranging from stigmatization to a wish for invisibility of this population, are pervasive and have great influence on the provision of necessary services. Nationwide efforts to sensitize the public in a positive way regarding the plight and needs of the mentally ill have been launched in the past by such influential figures as Dorothea Dix, Clifford Beers, and Rose Kennedy and most recently by Rosalynn Carter, but given the magnitude and prevalence of these detrimental attitudes, it is not surprising that such changes are difficult to effect. In the long run, however, such efforts are much more important than other change processes since they directly influence the acceptability of mental illness as a fundable medical condition and thus facilitate the provision of effective quality care for a huge segment of our population

PREREQUISITES FOR INSTITUTIONAL CHANGE

In the reports of the various efforts to change mental health institutions that have been published since 1969 several common themes emerge that may serve as guidelines for those considering the process of change in state mental hospitals.[5-10]

Support from Above

There is probably no single prerequisite for change as important as support from "above." Even if the changes contemplated are internal and entirely within one's preview and control, without the understanding and support of superiors in the department of mental hygiene they will be less than totally· successful. An example of this rule may involve support on something as seemingly indisputable as raising the quality of treatment plans or discharge plans, which may involve a temporary, but massive, redeployment of clinical and teaching staff. Unless departmental authorities realize the clinical as well as administrative and political importance of such an effort, it may be seen as a needless enterprise that siphons energy away from more important duties.

Active Leadership

The second most important ingredient in successful change efforts is an active leader. The selection of a person whose record has been that of maintenance and day-to-day steady managing to lead a change effort, obviously, will result in more of the same. It is surprising how often mental health services select persons to innovate who in the past have never originated or initiated any changes. Fairweather has noted that administrators with histories of job mobility are the most receptive to change processes.[6]

Critical Mass of Change Agents

Little can be accomplished if only a single individual is brought in to change a decrepit behemothic institution. There should be a sizable number of like-minded individuals who together can produce the expected innovations. What constitutes a "critical mass" of individuals varies with the size of the institution, its chronicity, its inclination to move with minimal effort, and its history of responsiveness to change. For instance, experience has shown that sending two newly trained policemen into a large precinct as a team dramatically increases their chances of surviving the inevitable socialization process imposed by older hands.[11] Other work has demonstrated that even the introduction of three key top administrators into a rigid system was not enough to alter it.[10] Change-agent teams or newly appointed directors of state hospitals in several instances have brought in a core group of 6 to 12 well-trained professionals with common beliefs and shared goals who have successfully turned around resistant systems.[7, 9, 12]

What is important for change agents in performing their mission is not to disregard any function or service. For instance, taking over administrative but not educational activities will lead to disaster. Controlling clinical but not business administration is equally unproductive.

Change-oriented individuals must be available throughout the entire system. While Fairweather comments on the necessity of importing persons from outside the system to bring about change, it is equally important to identify change-responsive persons within the system itself and convert them as quickly as possible to your aims. Their assistance is needed, not only to multiply the strength of the effort and to provide a communication system between innovators and hospital staff, but also to serve as a barometer of how improvements are proceeding.

A Clear Mandate

Important to the success of any change effort is the clarity of the charge given to the change agents and the acknowledged responsibility of the chief administrator for the objective. As has been described elsewhere,[13] if the message is "You do it, not me," the change agent will be undercut. If the upper echelons support the effort but will not provide a clear mandate, the effort is doomed. The proposers of innovation must make clear to the change agents and the recalcitrant institution that they are implementing a change process with a particular expectation. Thus in one state hospital after the director imposed new leadership on a deficient section of the hospital, he convened a hospital-wide meeting and explicitly stated that he expected the new staff head to bring his unit up to acceptable standards and expected such changes to have a halo effect throughout the rest of the hospital.[10]

The Right Time

Selecting the right time to begin a change process is also critical. Times of stability may seem more suitable for change than times of turmoil, but the energy available to move the institution is greater when there is a crisis and the chances of mobility are increased. This is especially true when the crisis is posed by an external threat to which the entire hospital system can respond. Then resentments and internal feuding are put aside to combat the outside force, and change becomes more likely. This phenomenon occurs very frequently during the hospital accreditation process. Today the threat of being disaccredited is very real. Internal crises also provide an opportune time to intervene, such as those precipitated by instances of patient abuse, a rash of suicidal or violent behavior, or incompetance effecting patient care. At such times the director or change agent has an ideal opportunity to unite the staff, work toward a common goal, and implement all sorts of innovations in the process.

The Right Place

Where one starts is as important as when one starts. If the area selected is the most resistant to change, difficulty or failure to bring about the intended result may doom further efforts. As an example, a change-agent team selected the geographic unit in a large state hospital most receptive to their presence and goals to begin a major effort of innovation. This unit was led by a resourceful and innovative leader, who had expressed curiosity about the team's functioning and collaborated with it on a previous project. Despite the immense difficulty of the team's task, it was immeasurably easier than working with a unit where the prognosis was poor. Success in the chosen area made the possibility of success at the next task more likely.

Sometimes one cannot pick an easy "winner," either because there is not one, or because the pressure of a crisis somewhere else requires action there. In this case careful assessment of success-enhancing factors is crucial. Such factors include staff favorable to the change effort, maximum utilization of change agents, comprehensive prediction of resistances, and utilization of every known person and technique.

Flexibility

Success at inducing or implementing change is enchanced by selecting an area amenable to change as evidenced by a previous record of flexibility and change. Oftentimes, even though specific innovations may be an anathema to a staff, their ability in the past to move, change, and respond in a flexible manner predicts their ability to do so again.

Open Communication

Opening up communication networks has a dramatic effect on the possibility of producing changes. Not only can the message of change be heard more clearly and more often, but feedback is more reliable, and the opening-loosening process has a halo effect of inducing others to open up and loosen up as well. Greenblatt[7] has suggested that encouraging "end-runs" and breaking up traditional lines of communication, frowned on by students of classical administrative theory, enhances and encourages the change process without significant danger. A predictable effect of opening communication in a hospital accustomed to rigidity and hierarchical control is suspicion concerning the hidden agenda behind this change. Inevitably, telling staff where one desires to make changes or encouraging participation in decision making and planning incurs a response of suspicion and distrust about what is hidden behind the overt statements. Such suspicion is only erased with time and the evidence of actual deeds.

Increasing Participation and Decreasing Central Authority

A corollary to open communication is the attempt to decrease reliance on centralized decision making when attempting to bring about change. All who will be affected by the process should be involved in the change efforts. Time and time again persons who have actively participated in change efforts have commented how successful this method of problem solving and decision making is.

By sharing the problems with the entire staff and fostering a group process aimed at finding solutions, the administration will not only have a plan of action that all should benefit from, but also will have a cooperative staff to carry out the proposals. The staff will also understand why the administration sought the changes, thus eliminating the we/they feeling of staff toward administration. In addition, the involvement of many people spreads the burden of responsibility, increases the chances of changes being accepted by another group, and increases the possibility of intentional or unintentional co-option of recalcitrant staff members.

Valuing Change Itself

The concept of the value of change in and of itself has both positive and negative aspects. Greenblatt[7] contends that such a view enhances the possibility of innovation. There is however, a danger of "the whirling dervish syndrome,"[13] where change for the sake of change may result in lateral or retrogressive change, not a change for the better. When successful, though, the encouragement of change, whatever its direction, does enhance loosening, creativity, and movement and may well be on the right path.

New Courses of Action—Not the Alteration
of Current Practices

Whenever possible, the utilization of new ideas, programs, staff or structures is preferable to the alteration of older elements. This is important because old and familiar networks and ideas carry the memories of the past and become difficult to use for new efforts. For example, two hospitals attempted to change their record keeping after years of following the same method and philosophy. One imported a new records librarian from outside the system to begin with the new program, whereas the other "recycled" an existing librarian through a training program. The first was very successful in putting the program into effect since to the outsider there was no other way, whereas, as committed as the second librarian was to the new changes, he kept remembering the previous policies and constantly had to translate the new into the old, like a newly learned foreign tongue. The danger of the dictum, "Find new, don't alter old," is that with entirely new ideas, programs, people, and administrative procedures and structures one has constant chaos without any stable elements. Since the problem with state hospitals is more often complete entropy and apathy rather than too much movement, it is difficult to become too innovative.

Changing Tactics

The chances of success for change efforts improve if the tactics used to achieve the goal are varied. For instance, while it is valuable to have staff visit another facility where an innovation has been successfully introduced (e.g., the use of problem-oriented records or the integration of sexes on wards), visitation may become a less useful learning experience if repeated too often, particularly if not reenforced by other techniques. Alternative methods of familiarizing staff with new programs may produce better results, such as lectures and demonstrations by visiting professors, preparing papers or project proposals on a desired innovation, refresher courses that cover new approaches in a particular service, in-service training, rotating students in training programs, or temporary participation by staff in programs in other facilities and then "education" by them of their colleagues on their return. No handbook of "how-to" tactics is available to the change-oriented administrator, but brainstorming with a group of like-minded peers, avid and wide reading in administrative journals, and familiarity with the basic bibliography presented at the end of this chapter will help one interested in initiating change.

Dissemination of Information

Part of the opening of communication has to do with the dissemination of information regarding the initiation or institution of changes. Publicity surrounding new developments that have had a desirable effect on quality of patient care and staff morale has the added effect of inducing such changes elsewhere. At one hospital the opening of a hotel ward designed to assist patients returning to community life to adjust to decreased staff attention and structured activities along with increased opportunities for self-reliance and independence, produced such a flurry of positive results that hospital staff elsewhere sought to replicate the program. Publicizing a successful innovation and how it works stresses the importance of change and often produces a halo effect just by its occurrence.

Attack on All Fronts

Greenblatt's efforts to change Boston State Hospital were successful in part because of his philosophy of attacking on different fronts at the same time.[7] If one can expend the staff and energy, it is clearly preferable to address clinical care, teaching programs, research, business administration, community relations, outreach facilities, and university affiliations simultaneously. Even if one has limited resources, not all efforts need large numbers of change agents and progress can proceed without direct intervention. For example, one director spent his energy and manpower on improving one area in the hospital, but at the same time he initiated a major review of all patients' discharge plans by the existing staff. Although they were apathetic and regid and resisted change, they were responsible and careful individuals. As the result of their review, they worked to improve deficiencies that they uncovered. They would not have done so had they not exposed the problems themselves.

Encouragement of More Change

Once changes have been made, there is an inclination to rest for a while. Whereas this may be possible in political campaigns or even military battles, it is not desirable in state hospitals. The magnitude of the job is so great that whatever the change, there are ten more tasks waiting, and part of the job of the change agent is to keep the process moving. Mao Tse-tung was aware of this on a societal level and advocated a new revolution every five years or so in order to prevent stagnation and rigidity. Luckily for the change-oriented individual in the state hospital, so long as he or she stays involved the press of new or unsolved problems is great enough to make his presence a continuing necessity.

THE FATE OF CHANGE AGENTS

In my estimation there are four positions that change agents occupy—or, to state this another way, four ways in which the system utilizes such persons to bring about changes. At the top are the commissioners of mental health and below them, at the institutional level are the directors or superintendents of state facilities. Two other types who may work either on a systemwide or at an institutional level are outside consultants and teams of change agents employed by the department of mental hygiene.

As long as the gratification resulting from the struggle to change an institution outweighs the frustrations, the commissioner, director, consultant, or team member is able to maintain a high energy level directed at changing the hospital or system for the better. There is a limit to everyone's endurance, however, and sooner or later the person who senses a shift in the balance and sees little chance of success will succumb to one or more of the following courses of action:

1. Adapting to the system
2. Being swallowed up by the system
3. "Burning out" early in the change process
4. Shifting the locus
5. Leaving the system

Having served in three of the four roles of change agents and observed closely several commissioners during their terms of service, I can attest that, regardless of the level, these have been the fates of most change agents.

Adaptating to the System

Some adaptations by change agents to the hospital or system are positive in that they permit the individual to use the forces inherent within the system to assist in changing it. In practice one more often sees negative adaptations, adaptations that seem destructive or counter to the change effort. In summarizing these I have used terms that are usually associated with individual defense mechanisms, adaptive reactions, and psychiatric syndromes. All refer only to the person's response to the change situation and are not necessarily part of the agent's character armor outside the work area.

Denial that there is anything to be concerned about is a common adaptive response. It is commonplace to hear directors of state facilities puzzling over charges made in the press or resulting from investigations as to staff incompetence, patient safety, or inadequate psychiatric treatment. They do not acknowledge their existence or fail to recognize the situations. Some administrators in the mental health system do isolate themselves from access to information and close their eyes to the patients walking about them. It is more common, though, for persons to see the damning evidence but fail to let it register cortically. Thus, despite statistics on patient injuries, misdiagnosis, lack of adequate community residences, etc., the official acts *as if* nothing were apparent or occult.

Projection, externalization, and displacement are all encountered frequently among administrators in the mental health system. While pure projection—"It's not me who's the culprit, it's you"— is widely found, far more common is externalization—"All my troubles come from those incompetents above." Whatever the change agent's initial orientation, it is inevitable that at some point, when frustrated by the lack of progress and movement, he or she will succumb to the notion that the problem is really out of his or her hands and the result of "those nitwits upstairs." Displacement usually accompanies the assignment of responsibility externally for one's problems. In addition to perceiving all one's troubles eminating from superiors, it is commonplace for people to assign responsibility or blame for the problem not to its origin but to a displaced object. Thus, officials will rail about the arbitrary and unjust standards by which accrediting bodies measure their staffing or treatment programs, rather than attack the sources of their difficulty—their own departments of mental health, their state legislature, or their own leadership abilities.

Isolation and insensitivity are reactions that characterize a certain breed of administrator who sees, registers and grasps the surrounding horrors but is not affected by them. This is usually the consequence of long service, prolonged exposure to the disasters, and a sense of defeat about coping successfully with difficulties. The resultant callousness, insensitivity, and seeming uncaring constitute a way of dealing with the recurrent pain of looking at the situation and knowing that easy solutions are not forthcoming.

A common adaptive mechanism is *withdrawal.* There can be withdrawal into other activities or oneself either of which removes the agent from the field of battle. People who resort to the first course of action disengage themselves from the struggle to change the hospital and divert their energies into university politics, research activities, their professional organization, or any number of activities or interests, which, while valid and needed, are not central to the goal of patient care in the institution. Withdrawal can also occur into oneself, a process whereby the administrator or consultant stops being concerned with changing external conditions and becomes self-occupied or engrossed with personal interests.

Rationalization is one of the most frequently encountered adaptive maneuvers of state hospital personnel. This approach ensures that one is never responsible for one's difficulties because "it's the same everywhere else," "no one else has been able to solve the problems," or "the whole thing is so out of my control that even thinking about it is futile." One director responded to a charge that the incidence of violent crimes was high inside his hospital by stating that it was the same as the crime rate in the community surrounding the hospital, thus obviating his need to remedy the situation.

Depression and despair result from the increasing sense of futility at remedying the situation in state facilities. This is frequently a spectrum phenomenon where the previous balance of gratification/frustration tilts first toward discouragement, then progresses to disillusionment, then despair, and finally hopelessness at ever remedying the conditions. Persons found on this spectrum appear beaten down, weary, and tired. They express a wish to be relieved of the burden, and while blaming no one but themselves for their plight, there is a strong tinge of masochism as well as triumph at surviving despite the odds.

Cynicism and anger are another set of adaptations frequently encountered. Here, the persons involved berate their superiors, convey the message that what else can one expect from such simpletons, and express the wish to get out of their positions—although they betray their true intentions by staying and complaining rather than leaving. The number of cynics in the state mental hospital system is astounding —most of them intelligent and formerly energetic individuals who now pour all their thinking and activity into fighting the system, castigating its administration, and derogating its structure.

Identification with the aggressor is encountered in persons who feel so put upon that the only way they can survive is to stop fighting and begin joining their perceived oppressors. Unfortunately, this adaptation carries with it the adoption of a role that is usually an exaggerated version of the truth. Thus the newly acquired behavior is worse than any real oppression encountered was. These individuals, previously so receptive to trying to alter the status quo, now become its primary defenders.

Concern with self-preservation becomes a preoccupation and even a way of life for many in the state system. Clearly, no one takes risks or attempts change processes if motivated primarily by the desire to stay alive in the system. In fact, those who are so predisposed, represent one of the major obstacles to change since anything that threatens the status quo and the calm progression of their careers is a danger to be dealt with.

Change as an end in itself, as mentioned earlier in this chapter, is a danger for change-oriented individuals. If an administrator becomes so enamored with the process and reality of *any* change, the substance of the change becomes secondary to its existence. Thus, for some individuals, the defense against grappling with substantive problems is to set a thousand moves in motion at the same time, each potentially canceling the other's effect. Just as the *process* of psychoanalysis may become a defense against analyzing so may the process of change defend against substantive change.

Being Swallowed Up by the System

If the change-oriented consultant or administrator lacks sufficient strength and vitality, finds insufficient support coming from superiors or peers, or is faced by a huge wall of bureaucratic and professional resistance, he or she may succumb to the system. Such giving up and giving in, while distressing to the onlooker, brings great relief to the sufferer. Time and again the system has proved that it is bigger than most of us. No matter how firm one's mandate, clearly spelled out the problems to be solved, or how realistic one is about the struggle ahead, the odds against success remain overwhelming in many systems and resignation to the inevitable occurs all too often, all too soon.

Early Burnout

The community psychiatric literature is replete with examples of energetic, change-minded, idealistic individuals who enter jobs with high hopes, work with tremendous energy, and burn out in a year or two.[14] This is equally true of administrators in the state mental hospital system. Many consultants, directors, and commissioners when they first come to a position fight valiantly for (in the history of the institution) a brief period and then burn out and turn to something else. Sometimes it is a job "upstairs," sometimes a flight into academic life or private practice, and sometimes a lateral move to a different state or locality under the impression that things are different elsewhere. Often there is the fantasy of return to the fray after a period of time, but more frequently there is the expressed wish never to return because of the toll such jobs take, the small amount of progress possible, given the amount of energy expended, and the sense of relief both at being out of the firing line and back with ones family, friends, and peers in a safer world.

Shifting the Locus

It is characteristic of change-minded individuals that they shift the locus of battle or level of struggle after encountering resistance or defeat. While some activists give up or keep on fighting after running into a wall, more often the response is to shift the field of action, switch tactics, or move to a new location or job to attack the problem afresh. It is not unusual to hear a change-oriented individual describe his moves from administration to consultation to another level of administration and so forth. Some proceed up the administrative ladder under an increasingly pressured fantasy that, given a high enough vantage and a powerful enough position, they can accomplish the job. Others move back and forth between line and staff positions, between consulting as a change agent and administrating as one, between direct involvement in the battle and supervising the strategy from afar in their attempt to accomplish their ultimate objective.

Leaving the System

Inevitably all change agents and administrators leave the system. Only a few senior people leave at retirement age, most leave long before. A few change-oriented individuals leave the moment their efforts are frustrated. Most, however, do not give up immediately; they go through adaptive phases, lateral moves, and attempts to alter the system from different vantage points before exiting. Ulett, in 1970, surveyed the length of time commissioners of mental health departments stayed in that particular job and found that the average was 5.4 years.[15] Informal samplings of state hospital directors has revealed an even lower figure among this group and a still lower average among consultants and consulting teams. It is interesting to learn the reason behind an individual's decision to leave the system altogether. There seems to be some internal balance that shifts, much as the gratification/

frustration balance mentioned before shifts, and with the shift a "click" is heard, like that described by alcoholics who pass a point of narcotization. At this point the decision is made that it no longer is worth the effort. In my informal soundings of individuals who have made the decision to leave, the reasons and precipitants are not at all clear, but the feeling of the need to move on is absolutely clear. As one change agent described it, "It was just like coming about in a sailboat; you didn't know how long it took, but you knew exactly when it was, and there was no turning back."

RESISTANCES TO CHANGE

There are literally dozens of types of resistance encountered in the change effort, many of which have been discussed in Chapters 2 through 4 regarding history, listed in Chapter 5 as constraints, and referred to in Chapter 8 as previous change efforts. In this section only a few resistances, most of which have been highlighted in the litera- ture, will be discussed and their phenomenology and possible ways to deal with them considered.

Personal Passive Aggressivity

Probably the most common resistance encountered by anyone working in any system is that of the passive-aggressive individual. Here there is no organized revolt or choreographed resistance, but rather an attempt by a single small cog in the system to maintain autonomy not by fostering change but by resisting it while appearing to cooperate with the process. Since it is usually impossible to fire such persons, since they have achieved a status, rank and familiarity within the system that ensures their survival, it is best to quickly identify them, actively co-opt them, use their seeming acceptance of change to give credential to the changes or to vitiate whatever influence they have by putting them out to pasture or into staff positions lacking the authority to block or hinder proposed moves.

The Reluctance of All Human Beings to Change

Not so much resistance as reluctance characterizes the response of all human beings to changes affecting their lives. The only way to counter this inherent characteristic is to give both verbal and then realistic assurances rather than merely state that the new way will make some parts of people's lives easier. Such assurances must materialize, of course, or they can be used only once, since staff members will not be receptive the next time. For example, unit personnel may be reluctant to directly participate in the admission process of patients, arguing that it will take them from pressing unit duties. However, if it can be shown that as a result their participation will speed up the initial evaluation and obviate repetitions in examinations and procedures—they may be more willing to try out the new process.

Organized Staff Resistance

Another obstacle usually encountered when trying to innovate is organized resistance on the part of many staff members to changing their ways. Greenblatt[7] has advocated shaking up the staff through the infusion of new ideas and concepts, and the Giordanos[16] mention the importance of spreading decision-making powers among the staff to encourage their participation in the change process and thus break down their resistance. Active and undisguised co-option through massive participation, involvement of the leaders of the resistance, and personal contact with pockets of resistance helps greatly too. The long-understood effect that personal contact and mutual respect have in mediating differences of opinion is essential to use. Just as it is very difficult in war to shoot the man whose face you can see, it is difficult to oppose the administrator whose goals and courage you know and respect. Such familiarity and contact take time to nurture, but they pay off handsomely.

Inflexible and Segmented Administrative Structures

A rigid or compartmentalized organizational structure is a sizable counterforce for any change agent to overcome. To combat this, two maneuvers are helpful: (1) opening up communications as much as possible[5] and broadening those lines that already exist and (2) making the structure less autocratic and more participatory.[16] Opening, flattening, and broadening moves all enhance the change process and reciprocally, decrease resistance.

Unclear Goals

To combat the resistance posed by unclear goals, it is necessary to clarify guidelines and programs.[5] Much time is spent by resistant staff members on demanding a clarification of where "this" is all leading to.

Too frequently their cause is aided by the ambiguous, vague, and ill-defined explanation of the goals sent from the top down.

System Resistance

The most prominent system resistance in the state mental hospital is in changing from custodial care to active treatment and rehabilitation. Aside from the realistic problems (e.g., lack of an effective technology, overwhelming nature of chronic mental illness, inadequate in-hospital and community resources) there is also the more global push for retention of the custodial care system. As Fowlkes[3] has demonstrated, this pressure from society, the professions, and the mental health system itself for retention of its traditional custodial role by state hospitals is overwhelming evidence of our wish to keep things as they are. The only effective solution to this problem is by changing the total direction of this shared wish at its source (the citizenry), not at its end-organ (the hospital).

A BASIC BIBLIOGRAPHY FOR CHANGE AGENTS OF STATE HOSPITALS

Since the general books on administrative theory provide inadequate preparation for the task of altering the state hospital situation, the change-oriented individual must complement these texts with a list that is broader, more radical, and more imaginative. The following represents a beginning basic bibliography:

1. Alinsky, Saul D. *Reveille for Radicals.* New York, Vintage Books, 1946.
2. Alinsky, Saul D. *Rules for Radicals.* New York, Random House, 1971.
3. Aquarius, Qass. *The Corporate Prince: A Handbook of Administrative Tactics.* New York, Van Nostrand Reinhold, 1971.
4. Clausewitz, Carl von. *On War.* New York, Penguin Books, 1968 (originally 1832).
5. Haley, J. *The Power Tactics of Jesus Christ.* New York, Discus/Avon, 1969.
6. Jay, Anthony. *Management and Machiavelli.* New York, Bantam, 1968.
7. Machiavelli, N. *The Prince and Other Discourses.* New York, Modern Library, 1940.

8.   Mao Tse-tung. *On Guerrilla Welfare*. New York, Praeger, 1961.
9.   O.M. Collective. *The Organizers Manual*. New York, Bantam, 1971.
10. Townsend, R. *Up the Organization*. Greenwich, Conn., Fawcett, 1970.

REFERENCES

1.   Golembiewski RT: Organization development in public agencies: Perspectives on theory and practice. Pub Admin Rev 29:4, 1969
2.   Feldman S, Cahill PA: Educating the mental health administrator: A report. Admin Ment Health 3:86–89, 1975
3.   Fowlkes MR: Business as usual—at the state mental hospital. Psychiatry 38:55–64, 1975
4.   Lawrence PR, Lorsch JW: Organization and Environment. Homewood, Ill., Irwin, 1969
5.   Kaplan HM, Balin D: Organizational obstacles to change in a large mental hospital. Am J Psychiatry 126:1107–1114, 1970
6.   Fairweather, GW, as cited in Hospitals' resistance to change probed in NIMH research, Psychiatric News, January 3, 1973, p 9
7.   Greenblatt M, Sharaf MR, Stone EM: Dynamics of Institutional Change: The Hospital in Transition. Pittsburgh, University of Pittsburgh Press, 1971
8.   Schulman J: Remaking an Organization: Innovation in a Specialized Psychiatric Hospital. Albany, State University of New York Press, 1969
9.   Seitz PFD, Jacob E, Koenig H, Koenig R, et al: The Manpower Problem in Mental Hospitals: A Consultant Approach. New York, International Universities Press, 1976
10. Talbott JA, Goodman P, Shapiro N, et al: Administrative receivership and troika management. Admin Ment Health 4:17–28, 1977
11. Talbott JA, Talbott SW: Training police in community relations and urban problems. Am J Psychiatry 127: 894–900, 1971
12. Talbott JA: The Para-professional teaches the professional. Am J Psychiatry 130: 805–808, 1973
13. Talbott JA, Keill SL: A typology of state hospital directors. Unpublished manuscript
14. Freudenberger HJ: The staff burn-out syndrome in alternative institutions. Psychother 12:73–82, 1975
15. Ulett GA, Schnibbe H, Ganser LJ, Thompson WA: Mental health director: Bird of passage. Am J Psychiatry 127:1550–1554, 1971
16. Giordano J, Giordano G: Overcoming resistance to change in custodial institutions. Hosp Community Psychiatry 23:183–185, 1972

10
What Has Been Tried

In their review of the literature Seitz and his associates isolated seven problems common to state hospitals. (1) largeness and isolation, (2) the strictures imposed by the hospitals' organization and functioning, (3) monolithic authoritarian administrative structures, (4) interdisciplinary communication and collaboration, (5) manpower shortages (numbers and skills), (6) weakness of clinical leadership, and (7) custodial rather than active treatment orientation.[1] Several innovations have been introduced in recent years in an attempt to handle these problems, individually and collectively. These can be divided into four broad areas: administrative changes, changes in the role of state hospitals, changes involving the staffs of state facilities, and system changes.

Administrative Changes

The most prominent changes have taken place in the administrative organization and functioning of state hospitals. Although there is considerable overlap, these developments can be separated into four areas—decentralization, geographical responsibility, unitization, and modern management techniques.

Decentralization

Because of their huge size, distance from urban areas, lack of continuity of treatment, neglect of the chronic mental patient, general low level of care, lack of individual attention and treatment, and authoritarian monolithic administrative structures, state hospitals have eagerly embraced the concept of decentralization of administration. This development, pioneered in the early 1950s,[2] has been almost universally adopted by most states and state facilities. Decentralization allows the breakup of large institutions into several smaller organizations, each with its own administration; decision making occurs at a level where staff knows the most about patients and their programs,[3] and evaluation, treatment, discharge, aftercare, and readmission can all be done by the same staff familiar with a cohort of patients. The result is heightened morale, responsibility, and autonomy. Training possibilities are enhanced because a small integrated unit is involved.

To anyone who remembers the old state hospital, the new decentralized system represents a dramatic departure. Not so long ago diagnoses were established not by persons treating the patients—but by administrators at "staffing conferences." Decisions about home visits and time of discharge were made by a central, seemingly unrelated, senior psychiatrist with no day-to-day contact with the patient. Under decentralization there are a number of minihospitals housed in a larger structure—each with its own leadership, clinical arm, and power to make appropriate clinical decisions, and each held accountable for actions taken. Because the same, single staff of a minihospital is responsible for a cohort of patients, they see the patient for screening, admission, treatment, discharge, follow-up, and readmission or other necessary treatment.

As a result of consolidation of staff, it is impossible to perpetuate the sort of isolation between staff members that had existed when, in some hospitals, physicians had offices off the wards and made rounds once a day, social workers toiled away in their set of offices in the basement, and activities therapists saw patients in separate areas, from which they rarely moved. Now all tend to work in the same area, either on the ward with their patients or near it. A sense of teamwork is generally the constructive end result.

Staff training no longer consists of lecturelike teaching sessions with large numbers in attendance. It is now possible with a small group of staff, responsible for a single group of patients. Most hospitals took advantage of the shift to decentralization to emphasize team training rather than discipline-oriented training, supervision rather than didactic teaching, and patient-involved training rather than conceptual or issue-oriented training.

The problems encountered by decentralization are numerous. Most involve the resistance to any change by a staff used to an established structure and set of procedures. In addition, administrators, accustomed to tight control and centralized decision making, sometimes themselves resisted the shift to semiautonomous administrative structures. Others in the system who sensed a loss of power fought equally hard. Most threatened among these were the chiefs of disciplines (nursing, social service, psychology, activities therapy, etc.) who no longer controlled budgets and staffs of considerable consequence and whose roles were changed to staff positions with primary responsibility for quality of their discipline members, teaching, and consulting.[4,5] There was resistance as well from those acquiring more power or responsibility. At times lower level staff did not want to be required to make decisions, take responsibility, and be held accountable. Another problem was that of finding a sufficient number of competent middle managers to administer these autonomous minihospitals. Especially in institutions long accustomed to central decision making, finding persons with a familiarity with administration, budgeting, staffing, and clinical supervision was not always easy. In addition, staffing, while unified under a minihospital, becomes stretched much thinner than when there are huge numbers of staff to draw on in case of sickness, emergency, etc., in one area. This is most evident if hospitals mix acute and chronic patients. In this instance, the resultant mixture of staff reveals how woefully understaffed "back-wards" were.

The organization of minihospitals varies. While most moved toward a geographic orientation—that is, Minihospital A took responsibility for County X or neighborhoods in the northeast sector of the city —many hospitals moved toward specialized or functional units, e.g., units that handled geriatric, alcoholic, adolescent, borderline mentally retarded, or violent/criminal patients. The move toward geographic unitization was the most prevalent in state hospitals until the recent past and will be discussed next.

Geographic Responsibility

As health planners became more concerned with the chaotic state of governmental hospitals, and spurred by the development of community psychiatry and community mental health centers, state hospitals were assigned specific geographic responsibilities. At one time six gigantic state hospitals 50 to 60 miles from New York City acted as an overflow for the mentally ill from the city who could not be handled locally. State planners halted the indiscriminate referral of patients, miles from their homes, neighborhoods, and neighbors, and each was given a specific geographic area of responsibility. The logical consequence was not only an assigned geographic responsibility, but also a breakup of responsibility so that patients from a given town, city, region, or even neighborhood were housed on the same ward. Often the geographic distinctions were arbitrary, as many such boundaries are, but the thrust was to group patients in a logical way, by area of origin, rather than acuteness or chronicity of illness. Patients were thereby mixed, there was an end to back-wards, and a hoped-for improvement by exposing chronic patients to those suffering from acute illness was frequently noted.[6] There was also an enhancement of the possibility that a single ward staff could know and relate to a small and graspable number of community agencies and facilities. No longer was the social worker at Manhattan State Hospital expected to know all 600 plus pages of the listing of agencies in Manhattan, while he or she could relate to not more than one-tenth that many.

In addition, geographic rather acute/chronic groupings necessitated the development of comprehensive services. No longer were active therapies present only on admissions and acute services, nor low-level occupational therapies clustered on the backwards, but all wards offered acute services, active treatment, rehabilitation, social services, etc. Responsibility for a single area offered a much greater possibility for relocating patients back into their communities than had the huge areas of service that most state hospitals had related to in past.

There are several problems, however, with the geographic housing of patients in a state hospital. Foremost among them is the fact that in hospitals serving large urban areas people move frequently and many patients are undomiciled. Catchment area lines, therefore, are limiting rather than facilitating, and readmission to a particular ward is often based on address rather than staff-patient familiarity. In addition, the formation of rigid boundaries sometimes leads to the "that's-not-my-table" phenomenon, where competition and buck-passing result in poor patient care. Another problem is that with the mixing of patients of all ages, diagnoses, and stages of activity and chronicity there is a mixing of poorly and less-poorly staffed wards, often resulting in a lower staff–patient ratio than is optimal.

Unitization

With geographic unitization the features of administrative decentralization and geographic responsibility are blended together. Geographic units have both the features described above—of autonomy, decentralized decision making, and clinical responsibility for a cohort of patients—as well as geographical relatedness to a particular community with all of the responsibilities and opportunities entailed.

The pioneering attempts at geographic unitization conducted in both Kansas and Duchess County, N.Y., have served as models for this development throughout the county.[7, 8] Recently, however, there have been increasing suggestions that hospitals move away from strict adherence to pure geographic unitization toward some specialized units (e.g., for adolescents, alcoholics, geriatric patients, etc.). Many hospitals, especially those that are part of the Veterans Administration, have found this organization useful.[9,10]

Modern Management Techniques

Utilizing Seitz et al's categorization of problems in state hospitals,[1] one is struck by the preponderance of issues related to administration or management—problems with the state hospital's social system, organization, functioning, administrative structure, communication, and collaboration. Smith and King[11] pointed out in another study of state facilities a similar list of problems, including goals, coordination, policy formulation, decision making, and change processes. It is no wonder, then, that many critics and observers of the mental health scene have suggested increased attention to modern management techniques and that the psychiatric literature makes increasing reference to authorities of management techniques.

Predictably, the techniques suggested range from "loosening," or creative, methods such as brainstorming, gaming, and T-groups to "tightening" mechanisms such as MBO (Managing by Objectives), cost-effectiveness analyses, and critical-path systems. In addition, consultation and direction have been sought from experts in human relations, organizational development, and operations research.

At present there is a hopefully creative tension between those we believe that nonmedical administrators should be more prominent in running mental hospitals and those who advocate more training in administration for clinicians.[12, 13] The American Psychiatric Association's Commission on Certification in Administrative Psychiatry has certified over 700 psychiatric administrators in the last 25 years, and for this certification administrative theory is required in addition to the traditional areas of personnel, budget, maintenance, etc. This gives proof to the strength of the movement to utilize more modern managerial practices in the mental health field.

CHANGES IN THE ROLE OF STATE HOSPITALS

The roles of state hospitals have also been changing dramatically in the recent past. In some instances their role has narrowed, in some it has broadened, and somewhat paradoxically it has occasionally moved in both directions at the same time. In addition, state facilities have undertaken several new programs to meet their changing needs and mandates.

Narrowing Their Tasks

Internal administrative decisions have changed the character of the population to be cared for by the state hospitals. These decisions specifically delineate which patients to admit and treat, thereby altering the role of the hospital. Its role has also been modified by the development of new or expanded mental health services in the community. Thus, these two forces—one internal, the other external—have narrowed the tasks performed by state institutions.

Probably the most dramatic example of an administrative change that affected the role of state facilities, occurred in New York in 1968, following a directive from the state commissioner's office. Facility superintendents were instructed to cease admitting patients not in need of acute psychiatric services—e.g., geriatric patients, persons with stable organic mental syndromes, or those ex-patients without adequate housing.[14] Since there had been no prior discussion with county, city, or local mental heath planners or providers and no alternative services for this population, the precipitate narrowing of the role of the state hospital produced an immediate and predictable crisis in the mental health system.[15] Other states have narrowed the tasks performed by state hospitals in much the same direction. They usually exclude those not in need of psychiatric treatment that would result in improvement of their condition—e.g., those in need of care not treatment, those in need of custody or asylum not therapy, and those for whom there are no alternative places to live.

The outside mental health facilities that have altered the role and tasks performed by state hospitals include private hospitals, outpatient clinics, child guidance clinics, psychopathic hospitals, general hospital inpatient and emergency services, and most recently, community mental health centers. The establishment of a nationwide network of community centers was intended to shift the locus of care from the outmoded state facilities to multiservice community facilities. In some cases this has happened, but reports are conflicting and mixed as to whether there facilities are really fulfilling their envisoned roles. Wolford and his associates report that in Pittsburgh their CMHC did bring about "lower rates of admission to the state hospital and decreased chronic hospitalization."[16] Such a trend therefore, has a direct effect on the population now served by the state facility and the services needed. Other reports demonstrate a trend in the opposite direction; for example, while total admissions may have decreased, the number of "patients with psychotic disorders and organic brain syndromes" was higher than expected.[17] In these instances the shift in types of patients served also necessitates a shift in the types of services provided by the state facility and narrows its functions.

Narrowing their task would logically seem to be a direction that would be welcomed by overburdened state hospitals. Whether the change emanates from an internal administrative shift or an external initiation of new services, if it is not accompanied by planning and flexibility to alter hospital resources, it may actually create more problems than it solves. Hospitals may be unable to shift their resources, change the mix of their staffs, or develop new programs to meet the new or altered demands of their population.

Broadening the State Hospital's Role

There has also been a trend toward broadening the role and functioning of state facilities. The two most popular models in recent years for such an expansion have been the community mental health center (CMHC) model and the human services model.

In the CMHC model the state facility has attempted to move in the direction of diversifying its services—moving from inpatient and some outpatient aftercare services—toward a panoply of services mandated by federal CHMC legislation. Under this legislation a facility provides inpatient, outpatient, partial hospital (day, night, and weekend hospital), 24-hour emergency and crisis, and community consultation and education services. At times this has been a pleasant change following the decrease in the census of hospitals that implement de-institutionalization and also acquire a geographically focused responsibility. Some state hospitals are too ambitious and take on more responsibilities than they can handle, e.g., expanding their role to serve alcoholics and drug abusers, children, etc. Other hospitals follow the CHMC model inflexibly, e.g., setting up separate partial hospital programs where they might better be integrated into existing hospital services. In this case personnel and support services may become stretched too thin and may duplicate other services in the community. Such a facility may lose the opportunity presented by the rundown in census, to increase staffing and quality and may have merely replaced one poor quality service with several. On the other hand, where diversification has worked, even on the ward level,[18] it offers hope for the future role of state facilities.

The human services model[19, 20] is not a fixed model such as the CMHC, with its mandated services. Its structure is based on the concept of the acquisition of a role of responsive interaction with community needs to fill in the apparent gaps in services. In other words, while the services needed might be those of the CMHC model (e.g., day hospital, aftercare, alcoholism, geriatric, support services) their creation and composition depends on what exists in the community and what is needed rather than duplication of services already present or creation of services not needed. The theory, while laudable, is based on the assumption that state facilities are flexible and adaptable enough to be sensitive to, respond to, and interact with community services and needs. It is questionable whether they are and whether, given the current climate of competition and distrust between elements in the mental health system, such a climate of cooperation is realistic. In addition, it opens state facilities to the role they have been trying desperately to avoid—becoming the filler of gaps, the provider of services no one else wishes to provide, in other words, the mental health services of last resort.

Initiating New Programs

The literature is replete with descriptions of new programs started by state facilities in recent years.[1, 21-25] This discussion is not concerned with the reasons behind the initiation of such programs but the content of such programs. They group logically into four areas: inpatient, transitional, aftercare, and community services.

Among these, inpatient programs have received the greatest attention. Most programmatic changes have involved a move toward therapeutic communities or therapeutic milieus. There are also numerous descriptions of the development of services involving group therapy, ward government, behavior therapy, geriatric services, and family therapy and family involvement.

Transitional services, designed either to assist patients in their return to full community functioning or to fill gaps in what is generally agreed should be a stepwise range of services from inpatient care to independent living, have received widespread attention, despite their continued meager number compared to their need. Such services include quarterway services, halfway houses, lodges, group living arrangements, communal apartments, foster homes, and programs specifically designed to prepare chronic patients to reassume independent functioning after years of dependent custodial care.[26] It is important to emphasize (1) that, given the results of de-institutionalization, many of these efforts come too late, in too few numbers and (2) that the task of prepairing patients for a return to the community has to begin in the hospital. It is no longer tenable to wait to see if patients will survive in welfare hotels or nursing homes before instituting reentry preparation programs.

Aftercare, which has also been too little, too late, is another area of increasing attention in recent years, especially concerning those patients who "drop through the cracks." Traditional aftercare services, which have been the province of understaffed, overextended state hospitals, have not provided the continuity of care, intelligent and diligent follow-up, and provision of needed outpatient services, required by chronic mental patients. Most lacking has been careful attention to maintaining patients in treatment rather than being mostly concerned about the existence of programs.[27]

Lastly, state hospitals have attempted to meet the needs of their discharged patients by establishing and expanding their community services. These include alternatives to inpatient care, partial hospitalization programs, emergency services and crisis intervention, and community support systems to enable patients to remain in the community. It cannot be overemphasized that as critical as these have been, sufficient alternatives have not been set up even to begin to fill the need of the large number of persons discharged from state hospitals in the past 20 years. The literature does have accounts of worthy programs, but these represent the rare and unusual rather than the commonplace and available, a problem which no one has yet solved.

STAFFS OF STATE HOSPITALS

Since the staffs of facilities are at the same time part of the problem of what to do with state hospitals as well as its solution, much effort and money has been expended on them in recent years. It is generally acknowledged that merely raising salaries does little to solve the problems faced by state hospitals, since in the past that approach has not attracted a substantially different quality staff. Instead, efforts have been made to form staff members into therapeutic teams, to train and retrain them, and to open hospital staff privileges to practitioners from the community.

Therapeutic Teams

Without question, one of the most popular, misunderstood, and abused innovations in recent times has been that of the formation of therapeutic teams to care for patients, whether on an inpatient or outpatient basis. In the past members of different disciplines went their own way, devised their separate treatments, and communicated for information purposes only. The intention of the teams of today is to encourage working together to maximize the information, skills, and therapeutic leverage possible. Geographic unitization, indeed any type of decentralization, coupled with moving professional staff to wards, engendered a team approach, and such developments as the interdisciplinary treatment plan, the requirement for continuity of care, and more thoughtful planning for discharge, furthered this team method.[28-30]

In theory, teamwork multiplies one's strength by putting into practice the dictum that "two heads are better than one," but for many state hospital staffs this just does not apply. Teams cannot be leaderless, and yet the assumption underlying many clinical teams is that all members are equal, regardless of legal responsibility, training, or expertise.[31] The abuses of teams have included voting (one man, one vote) on whether to discharge suicidal patients, seizing decision making by discipline majority or coalition, and becoming so involved in discussions and team meetings that little therapeutic work is possible. In addition, in some states where social workers and psychologists tend to be American-born and trained and physicians tend to be foreign-born and trained, the fight between nonphysicians and physicians has disrupted patient care at worst and silenced uncombative psychiatrists at best. Where nonphysicians assume the role of team leader, there is further opportunity for conflict.[32]

The discussion here does not mean to imply that teams cannot function more effectively than individuals going their own way, but the mere use of the word "team" for an interdisciplinary group of staff members working with patients does not guarantee better patient care. Only with carefully delineated roles for team members, both in a generic and specific discipline function, with persons willing to discuss and argue and then accept the leader's decision, and with adequate training available for all members of teams can an interdisciplinary team work. These are conditions rarely found in state hospitals.

Training

Since the mid 1960s a concertred effort has been made to upgrade training efforts in state facilities. This has occurred in three directions: to train paraprofessionals, to train interdisciplinary treatment teams, and to retrain staff for community activities.

With the introduction of geographic unitization and interdisciplinary treatment teams, nursing aides have become obsolete. They have been replaced by paraprofessionals. This change in name implies both an upgrading to engender working *alongside* professionals as well as a move away from custodial activities implied by the term aide or attendant toward a therapeutic role (intended by the word paraprofessional). Such a shift requires considerable training efforts. These have been well documented in the literature.[33, 34] Most have floundered on the difficulty in teaching a generic skill rather than merely training pseudopsychiatrists or social workers or on translating the sorts of education and training provided mental health professionals to paraprofessionals. Another difficulty has been in bridging work and classroom situations. The apprenticeship experience, provided to all mental health professionals in training in settings in which they will not necessarily be working, encourages them to learn, make mistakes, and grow. This is lacking in most paraprofessional training. Supervision, so essential to the education of professionals, is sometimes completely omitted with paraprofessionals, widening the gap between classroom instruction and the real life on state hospital wards.

One method of combating these gaps has been the development of interdisciplinary training teams who, in turn, consult with interdisciplinary treatment teams. Here, with competent trainers, skilled in clinical areas, and comfortable with each other, one may see the effective transfer of team skills and cooperation as well as didactic knowledge.[1, 35] Such work is exhausting, since the trainers must themselves function effectively as a team, and much time is spent on "team hygiene," team cross-training, and like disciplines training each other. While the dangers of burnout and theft by clinical elements in the system are always present, the thrill and productivity inherent in working with such a group makes the experience a rewarding one. Results of such training efforts are, however, less tangible, and it will be years before we know whether the millions spent on team training efforts in state hospitals have produced better patient care and better patient outcomes or merely raised expectations and frustrated ambitions for the majority of former state hospital attendants.

The last area of training to be utilized extensively in the recent past involves the retraining of existing inpatient staff to perform outpatient or community activities. As state hospitals have attempted to diversify their programs, either to meet new needs or to serve their deinstitutionalized ex-patients, they have frequently attempted to retrain staffs to function in new (community) roles.[36, 37] Such retraining is expensive, extensive, and comprehensive if it is to be effective. Like paraprofessional training, it must remove the trainee from familiar environment and place him or her in an optimal clinical and learning setting, like that where he or she will function in the future. The resistance to moving into new roles or locales is nowhere more apparent than here. The staff, long accustomed to custodial and moderately expectable tasks, is suddenly confronted with the strange, unexpected, and wide-open situation. Civil service unions have participated, sometimes reluctantly, in such efforts. The future of large shifts in the numbers of inpatient staff members to outpatient responsibilities will depend in large part on these unions' ability to persuade their members that community jobs lead to more career flexibility and growth than standard inpatient positions.

Opening Staffs

There has not been a widespread move toward opening state hospital staffs to professionals in the community. Such efforts deserve attention, however, for this approach may well lead to improved care and community acceptance faster than any other method.[38] When closed medical staffs are opened to psychiatrists and general physicians practicing in the nearby community, a more diversified medical staff is achieved, frequently with more status and community acceptance than the stereotypic state hospital medical staff. Consequently, inpatients and hospital staff see different models and methods of treatment, and community physicians see the insides of state facilities and have a better understanding of their strengths and weaknesses. Such a cross-fertilization may be an important ingredient for change if such is ever to occur.

SYSTEM CHANGES

All the previously discussed innovations occuring in state facilities essentially involve only the state facilities themselves. As such they are small steps in comparison with the task of changing the entire mental health system. Clearly, to effect substantive change, innovations must involve this entire system. Several developments presage the steps necessary to alter the entire system, to provide quality care for the mentally ill, and to improve the lot of the chronic and severely mentally ill now housed in state hospitals.

Joint Planning

The first step in a systems approach to solving the problem of state facilities is the development of joint planning that involves local, municipal, or county, and state facilities and governments as well as consumers.[39] Such planning may be voluntary or legislatively mandated. Experience has shown that it has begun to decrease the mutual distrust, suspicion, and fighting between the elements mentioned and has increased cooperation and service coordination. In some instances it has resulted in multiple use of facilities, interagency consultation, and staff sharing.[40] A perceptible defect, however, is the dramatic increase in meetings, which seem at times to constitute a new industry, as well as a misuse of planning, which becomes an end in itself and thus a defense against acting to implement the plans so devised. In the latter instances planning means talking. When public officials are unable or unwilling to move to action, frustration results in subversion of the process, cynical regard for all participants, and a building level of anger.

Division of Labor or Territory

Joint planning and cooperation can result in a division of labor or territory between otherwise competing facilities. Traditionally, state facilities have treated more chronic patients with multiple admissions and local facilities acute patients on their first admission. Their roles most recently have blurred that distinction. In some cases, however, clarification of the division of labor is possible. In other cases either the state or local facility may take total responsibility for a geographic area, thus moving toward a CMHC model, dividing the territory rather than the task.

Coordination of Services

While liaison and cooperation between local and state services has a long and venerated past, and descriptions abound of such arrangements,[41] it is only recently that there have been attempts to provide formal administrative linkages between such services. In North Carolina utilization of 10 area boards and area directors, with responsibility for both local and state services, provided the mechanism to move from separate to unified services in each catchment area.[42] Likewise, in Arizona the appointment of a coordinating body of university-state-local and CMHC officers, along with a jointly appointed director of CMHC and county services, provided the linkage necessary to furnish a unified service.[43]

Statewide Unification of Services

It is only with the unification of services on a statewide basis, however, that control of all elements in the mental health system (with the exception of the VA hospitals) is achievable. Probably the best known model for such a unification is in California, where following the L-P-S (Lanterman-Petris-Short) legislation, unified planning, funding, and services were mandated.[44, 45] Counties took responsbility for screening and alternatives to hospitalization and aftercare, and to a great extent they controlled the system. Such a change was not without its problems. The new system cost more. For a while there was was the promise of saving money by closing all state hospitals, but time demonstrated the need for their continuance to serve a core population of the chronically ill as well as to serve special population groups, such as dangerous patients. Second, there were not enough community alternatives in place from the start. In New York, where a unified services bill has been law since 1973,[46] the funding formula was too unappealing to entice counties to "buy in." As a result, there has been almost no change in the system.

The Future of a Unified System

Whatever the problems encountered in California, New York, and Massachusetts, to mention the most cited cases, the indications are clear that a move toward a unified system of mental health care is in the offing. While further discussion of the role of the state facility in such a system will be postponed to a later chapter, it is worthwhile at this point to mention some of the ingredients necessary before truly unified services may be achieved.[47,48] To have a unified system, there must be a single system of care with tracking of patients throughout the system; there must be single funding and planning; there must be effective system of triage; and there must be a regional plan taking into consideration regional differences in population at risk, problems, and services available.

REFERENCES

1. Seitz FD, Jacob E, Koenig H, Koenig R, et al: The Manpower Problem in Mental Hospitals: A Consultant Team Approach. New York, International Universities Press, 1976
2. Garcia L: The Clarinda plan: An ecological approach to hospital organization. Ment Hosp 11:30–31, 1960
3. Cumming J, Cumming E: Ego and Milieu: Theory and Practice of Environmental Therapy. New York, Atherton, 1969
4. Kernberg OF, Appelbaum A: Resolving a crisis in the activities therapy department. Hosp Community Psychiatry 24:225–230, 1973
5. Equinozzi AM, Wood RC: A study on the effect of institutional decentralization on department head functioning in state institutions. Unpublished paper
6. Brice JA, Gonda HH: The impacy of unitization on long-term patients. Hosp Community Psychiatry 22:341–344, 1971
7. Zubowicz G: The "Kansas" plan: The change to a unit system. J Kans Med Soc 65:12–17, 1964
8. Bennett CL: The Dutchess County plan, in Milbank Memorial Fund: Decentralization of Psychiatric Services and Continuity of Care. New York, the Author 1962
9. Klett WG, Watson CG: The unit system: Current staff attitudes and future directions. Hosp Community Psychiatry 24:539–542, 1973
10. Ellsworth RB, Dickman HR, Maroney RJ: Characteristics of productive and unproductive unit systems in VA psychiatric hospitals. Hosp Community Psychiatry23:261–268, 1972
11. Smith CG, King JA: Mental Hospitals: A Study in Organizational Effectiveness. Lexington, Mass. Lexington Books, 1975
12. Sheffel I: Non-medical administrators: Colleagues not rivals. Hosp Community Psychiatry 18:129–134, 1967
13. Foley AR, Brodie HKH: The administrative process as an instrument of change. Hosp Community Psychiatry 20:1–8, 1969
14. Robbins E, Robbins L: Charge to the community: Some early effects of a state hospital system's change of policy. Am J Psychiatry 131:641–645, 1974
15. Reich R, Siegel L: Psychiatry under seige: The chronically mentally ill shuffle to oblivion. Psychiatr Ann 3:35–55, 1973
16. Wolford JA, Hitchock J, Ellison DL, et al: The effect on state hospitalization of a community mental health center/mental retardation center. Am J Psychiatry 129:202–206, 1972
17. Kentsmith DK, Menninger WW, Coyne L: A survey of state hospital admissions from an area served by a mental health center. Hosp Community Psychiatry 26:593–596, 1975
18. Johnson E, Crockett JT, Cumpton E, et al: Adopting new models for continuity of care: The ward as mini-mental-health-center. Hosp Community Psychiatry 26:601–604, 1975

19. Schulberg HC: The mental hospital in the era of human services. Hosp Community Psychiatry 24:467–472, 1973
20. McAtee OB, Zirkle GA: The evaluation of a state hospital into a human-services center. Hosp Community Psychiatry 25:381–382, 1974
21. Zusman J, Bertsch EF (eds): The Future Role of the State Hospital. Lexington, Mass. Lexington Books, 1975, chaps. 10–13
22. Wooley FR, Kane RL: Community aftercare of patients discharged from Utah State Hospital, a follow-up study. Hosp Community Psychiatry, 28: 114–118, 1977
23. Winston A, Pardes H, Papernik DS, Breslin L: Aftercare of psychiatric patients and its relation to rehospitalization, Hosp Community Psychiatry 28:118–121, 1977
24. Furedy R, Crowder M, Silvera F: Transitional care: A new approach to aftercare. Hosp Community Psychiatry 28:122–124, 1977
25. Milby, JB: A review of token economy treatment programs for psychiatric inpatients. Hosp Community Psychiatry 26:651–659, 1975
26. Test MA, Stein LI: Special living arrangements: A model for decision-making. Hosp Community Psychiatry 28:608–610, 1977
27. Talbott, JA: Stopping the revolving door: A study of readmissions to a state hospital. Psychiatr Q 48:159–168, 1974
28. Pepper B: The Team: A means of achieving continuty of care, in Dean A, Kraft AM, Pepper B (eds): The Social Setting of Mental Health. New York, Basic Books, 1976
29. Shapiro ER, Gudeman JE: Using the team concept to change a psychoanalytically oriented therapeutic community. Hosp Community Psychiatry 25:166–169, 1974
30. Birjandi PF, Sclafani MJ: An inter-disciplinary team approach to geriatric patient care. Hosp Community Psychiatry 24:777–778, 1973
31. Birger D, Plutchik R, Conte HR: The evolution and demise of a crisis intervention program in a state hospital. Hosp Community Psychiatry 25:675–677, 1974
32. Greiff SA, McDonald RD: Role relationships between non-physician treatment team leaders and team psychiatrists. Community Ment Health J 9:378–387, 1973
33. Fulton GS, Wallach HF, Gallo CL: Training mental health workers to better meet patient needs. Hosp Community Psychiatry 25:299–302, 1974
34. Mehr J: Evaluating non-traditional training for psychiatric aides. Hosp Community Psychiatry 22:315–318, 1971.
35. Talbott JA, Ross AM, Skerett AF, et al: The paraprofessional teaches the professional. Am J Psychiatry 130:805–808, 1973
36. Karls JM: Retraining hospital staff for work in community programs in California. Hosp Community Psychiatry 27:263–265, 1976
37. Stein LI, Test MA: Retraining hospital staff for work in a community program in Wisconsin. Hosp Community Psychiatry 27:266–268, 1976
38. McQueen R: Problems of coverting a state mental health hospital into an open-staff facility. Psychiatry 33:119–126, 1970

39. Talbott, JA: Developments in metropolitan state hospital services, in Zusman J, Bertsch EF (eds): The Future Role of the State Hospital. Lexington, Mass., Lexington Books, 1975

40. Snow HB, Blackburn DP: Unifying state hospital and local services to prevent or shorten hospitalization. Hosp Community Psychiatry 24:487–489, 1973

41. Frey H, Muller DJ: Community mental health center and state hospital collaboration through busing of twenty-four patients, in Beigel A, Levenson AI (eds): The Community Mental Health Center: Strategies and Programs. New York, Basic Books, 1972

42. Rollins RL, Stratas NE: The geographic unit as a phase in merging hospital and community programs. Hosp Community Psychiatry 25:379–860, 1974

43. Beigel A, Bower WH, Levenson AI: A unified system of care: Blueprint for the future. Am J Psychiatry 130:554–558, 1973

44. California's unified service plan, in the future role of the state hospital. Hosp Community Psychiatry 25:383–384 1974

45. Barter JT: Sacramento County's experience with community care. Hosp Community Psychiatry 26:587–589, 1975

46. Forstenzer HM, Miller AD: Unified services in New York State, in Zusman J, Bertsch EF (eds): The Future Role of the State Hospital. Lexington, Mass., Lexington Books, 1975

47. Smith DC, Jones TA, Coe JL: State mental health institutions in the next decade: Illusions and reality. Hosp Community Psychiatry 28:593–597, 1977

48. Stratas NE, Bernhardt DB, Elwell RN: The future of the state mental hospital: Developing a unified system of care. Hosp Community Psychiatry 28:598–600, 1977

PART IV

Solutions

11

The Range of Options

It should be obvious by now that state hospitals, as they are currently constituted, do not work, seem designed not to work, and have never worked. Whatever we are doing, we are not doing it right. Critics of the state mental hospital system continue to point out the problems, decade after decade, without any perceivable effect.[1-4]

Many activities of state facilities seem to be designed to avoid treating patients. For example, the preoccupation with paperwork, internal politics, civil service regulations, and such trivia as wearing white coats on duty seems to serve as defenses against facing the real and overwhelming tasks existing in the state system. The tasks thus avoided include (1) the public health responsibility—e.g., serving as the facility of last resort for the rest of the mental health system's frustrations and failures—and (2) the difficulty in treating and caring for the chronic mental patient. If these tasks were faced squarely, the state mental health system would have to admit (1) that it cannot assume this sweeping a public health responsibility given the reality of dumping, dangerous patients, the revolving door, etc., and (2) that chronic mental patients need both more stabilizing, continuous, long-term treatment and care and different staff, programs, and rehabilitation-focused treatment.

State mental hospital systems in recent years have attempted to restrict admissions and lower retentions (de-institutionalization) and then ultimately to close some hospitals as ways of running away from the dilemma of being confronted with the expectation of performing

125

these tasks without adequate social, moral, and financial support. The press and professionals, many of whom initially supported these moves, have begun to oppose this flight from responsibility. It was not, however, until such critics as Lamb and Goertzel[5] addressed themselves to the question of one real issue—care and treatment of the chronic patient—underlying these moves that grappling with substantive issues became possible.

Thus the problem remains. We have a huge mental hospital system —with buildings, employees, and patients. On the one hand, it is not working, and something needs to be done. On the other hand, someone needs to be responsible for the care and treatment of a patient population no one wants, for which, ironically, state hospitals were invented over a century ago.

What then are the options? In the succeeding chapters, four commonly discussed solutions for the state mental hospital system will be examined.

These range from the most conservative (keeping them as they are) to the most radical (closing them altogether). Between these two extremes are the options of a drastic overhaul of the existing system and a pragmatic change in the role and function of the state mental hospital. Finally, some general guidelines will be offered that are applicable to any proposed solution if there is to be any substantive change in the way we address the care and treatment of the problem patients no one wants to treat.

REFERENCES

1. Belknap I: Human Problems of a State Mental Hospital. New York, McGraw-Hill, 1956
2. Deutsch A: The Shame of the States. New York, Harcourt Brace, 1948
3. Greenblatt M, York RH, Brown EC: From Custodial to Therapeutic Patient Care in Mental Hospitals. New York, Russell Sage Foundation, 1955
4. Mendel WM: On the abolition of the psychiatric hospital, in Roberts LM, Greenfield NS, Miller MH (eds): Comprehensive Mental Health. Madison, University of Wisconsin Press, 1968
5. Lamb R, Goertzel V: The demise of the state mental hospital—premature obituary? Arch Gen Psychiatry 26:489–495, 1972

12

The Conservative Solution:
Keep State Hospitals as They Are

The most conservative solution to the problem of state mental hospitals is to maintain the status quo, continuing to do more of the same as before. A 1973–1974 national survey of commissioners of mental health,[1] showed, not surprisingly, that a "great majority" of states were not planning to close mental hospitals; rather they were going to "modernize and expand their mental health delivery systems" through such efforts as

1. Improvement of staff–patient ratios.
2. Elimination of inappropriate admissions.
3. Transfer (services) to other auspices.
4. Orientation toward the communities.
5. Development of alternatives to institutionalization.

In short, the commissioners were not planning any substantive changes; they would cling to their existing plans, which had already been discredited.

THE PROPOSAL

Very few persons in the mental health system openly advocate keeping state hospitals exactly as they are now. Instead, the argument is made to go slow in planning alternatives or phasing them out, to make modest changes to improve their functioning, or to change them in the same direction as has been attempted in the past two decades. By deed, however, retaining hospitals as they are is what a number of states are doing. With no substantive changes being initiated, with increasing budget cuts and policy restrictions, and with inattention to the major tasks facing the hospitals, the result is the same old system.

It is not simply the commissioners of mental health who favor a continuation of the status quo. Pioneers such as Maxwell Jones state that "the state hospitals system failed because it never had a chance to succeed."[2] Quen, in an article entitled "Learning from History,"[3] implores us not to close state hospitals before we see why their promise was not realized. The titles of several other publications draw our attention to this position—Kubie's "The Responsibility of the Medical Profession to Provide Hospital Treatment,"[4] Rachlin's "The Case Against Closing of State Hospitals,"[5] and Williams' "Are They Closing The Mental Hospitals Too Soon?[6] While none of the works cited advocate keeping state mental hospitals *exactly* as they are now, they do give backing and comfort to those who wish to continue "business as usual."[7]

THE PROS OF KEEPING STATE HOSPITALS

Two of the major arguments favoring keeping the present set up of the state hospital system are the benefits of the maintenance of the status quo and the avoidance of additional expenditures by the state. In addition, the conservative alternative avoids any disruption of a political, professional, or clinical nature; does not threaten any jobs; and maintains a pluralistic mental health system (private, quasi-public, and public). It also offers the promise of housing the chronically mentally ill and providing some sort of asylum, but the current drift of state hospital services makes this promise look less and less likely.

THE CONS

Despite the fact that continuing to expand and improve the system sounds a great deal like progress, since the system is deteriorating, this actually constitutes a regressive solution. If it is not working well now, more of the same will work even less well in the future. In fact, perpetuation of the system ensures that scandals will continue, that chronic patients will continue to be unserved, and that the revolving door will continue to swing.

In addition, maintenance of the existing two-or three-class system is not pluralism; it is discrimination. And it is discrimination not only against the poor and racial minorities, but also against those who have severe and chronic mental illnesses rather than acute and moderate conditions. There may well be a need for a two-class system—but it should be one that provides equally good treatment, rehabilitation, and care for either acutely or chronically ill patients, not active treatment for acutely ill patients and custodial care for chronic patients.

Most damning as an argument against perpetuation of the system as it now exists is that with slight "tinkering" and modest increased funding there will be no attempt to change our entire philosophy of addressing the treatment and care of the difficult patient and no opportunity of ever introducing a single, comprehensive, prospective approach to mental health services. As it has been argued in Chapter 10, it is only by such a systems approach that we can hope to comprehend and subsequently to grapple with this overwhelming problem.

CONCLUSIONS

Undoubtedly there is a need for residential care for a small core population of severely and/or chronically mentally ill. The enthusiasm in the 1950s and 1960s for emptying out and restricting admission to state mental hospitals has been tempered by the realization in the 1970s that these policies merely moved chronic mental patients "from the frying pan into the fire." The question of what percentage of the population needs some form of asylum is as yet unanswered, but it is addressed more sensibly now than before.[8-10] Whether the place for such asylum is a state-funded, state-operated mental hospital is another question that demands equal attention.

Despite the fact that the pendulum has indeed swung too far from asylum psychiatry toward abandonment of patients into the community, it has gone too far ever to retrench completely. Since the prevailing trend for state hospital services is to comprise an ever decreasing amount of the total mental health services delivered in this country,[11] it would be folly to advocate retention of the state mental hospital as such. Far more likely there will be a shift in the role or function of the state-funded facility toward more specialized populations, an alternative to be discussed in a subsequent chapter.

REFERENCES

1. Horizon House Institute: The Future Role of State Mental Hospitals: A National Survey of Planning and Program Trends. Philadelphia, the Author, 1975
2. Jones M: Community care for chronic mental patients: The need for a reassessment. Hosp Community Psychiatry 26:94–98, 1975
3. Quen JM: Learning from history. Psychiatr Ann 5:11–31, 1975
4. Kubie LS: The responsibility of the medical profession to provide hospital treatment, in Zusman J, Bertsch EF (eds): The Future Role of the State Hospital. Lexington, Mass., Lexington, 1975
5. Rachlin S: The case against closing of state hospitals, in Ahmed PI, Plog SC (eds): State Mental hospitals. New York, Plenum, 1976
6. Williams RM: Are they closing the mental hospitals too soon? Psychol Today, May 1977, pp 124–129
7. Fowlkes MR: Business as usual - at the state mental hospital. Psychiatry 38:55–65, 1975
8. Brill H: The future of the mental hospital and its patients. Psychiatr Ann 5:9–21, 1975
9. Orwin A: The mental hospital: A pattern for the future. Br J Psychiatry 113:857–864, 1967
10. Stewart DW: The future of the state mental hospital. Prosp Psychiatr Care: 13:120–122, 1975
11. Taube CA, Redick RW: Provisional Data on Patient Care Episodes in Mental Health Facilities, 1975. Statistical Note No 139. Rockville, Md. National Institute of Mental Health, 1977

13

The Reformist Solution: Drastic Alteration of State Hospitals

It is self-evident that reform movements engender mixed reactions. To some, reform movements are crusading, valiant, righteous efforts to remedy a corrupt or deteriorated situation. To others, they are superficial Bandaids that may actually prevent substantive change through the promise of small improvements. In this chapter reform is considered as a thorough change of the state mental hospital system, one that would address all of the problems encountered by state facilities. I am not referring to the responses of the state hospital system over the past 100 years, following the scandals exposed by politicans or the press, because clearly these have not resulted in any substantive change.

Genuine reform must take into consideration everything from altering the stultifying personnel policies under anachronistic civil service laws to changing public opinion regarding mental illness and the mentally ill. Perhaps this is much too ambitious to undertake—*but* it is not too ambitious to discuss, and this discussion, to the best of my knowledge has never been held.

The massiveness of the job that needs to be done can be grasped by remembering all of the problems detailed in Chapters 5 through 8, which include constraints, politics, mentalities, and structural obstacles. Each of the problems mentioned in these chapters must be addressed if reform is to be successful.

Assuredly, this solution, if done correctly, is the most expensive of all the options, and for this reason it will probably never be undertaken. It is much cheaper to either keep state hospitals as they are or close them. The option of genuine reform, however, deserves our attention, for if the functioning of state facilities is ever to be realized, they must be given the opportunity and tools with which to do the task. And as Jones and others have stated, they have never really been given a fair chance.[1]

THE PROPOSAL

A reformist proposal involves across-the-board reform of *all* elements that impede state hospitals from performing their missions. It includes systems, social, state governmental, departmental, and individual institutional factors as well as elements present in the mental health professions, the public, and the legislature. In short, it involves a complete rethinking, restructuring and redoing of the state mental hospital system.

AREAS TO BE REFORMED

The following discussion will consider only the most arresting areas of the state hospital system that need to be "overhauled."

Personnel Policy

One of the most important areas in need of change is personnel policy. Autonomy in hiring and firing, in competing with peer institutions for talent, and in modifying staffing to meet programatic needs are but a few of the reforms necessary. Critical to this autonomy is a cessation of the hospital system's reliance on civil service, indeed any rigid bureaucratic procedure, and a substitution of guidelines, monitoring, and accountability to allow for sensible and creative personnel policies on the institutional level.

Budgeting

Budgetary reform is equally important. Primary in this area is the initiation of flexible budgetary processes including the options to switch monies between personnel and other-than-personnel areas, to reallocate monies from inpatient to outpatient or other community activities, and to contract with private or nonprofit hospitals, services, or agencies when in the patient's or system's best interests. In addition, funding should be flexible enough to support adequately new and necessary programs. All of this flexibility must be accompanied by true accountability, not the reams of paper, months of delay, and multiple levels of review that characterize today's extant pseudo-accountability. Delay and incompetence are not accountability—neither is automatic nay saying.

Mentalities

The smooth running of state facilities cannot be accomplished if personnel retain the traditional hospital mentalities. On a departmental level, those clinging to outmoded attitudes such as the bureaucratic, object/person, and quantification mentalities must either be subject to some humane form of thought reform or sent to a suitable state agency (for example, highways, water supply) where their adherence to rigidity, rules, property, and numbers will be adaptive. They should be replaced by staff who are more interested in people, problem solving, creativity, and quality of care.

A similar housekeeping chore exists at the institutional level. Those who regard treatment of the mentally ill as a factory job, one to be undertaken by monitoring and policing rather than by treating, and whose principal wish is to survive in a no-win world might do well to be transferred to buildings and grounds or the computer center, leaving their jobs free to be filled by professionals interested in personal and professional growth, in active involvement with the mentally ill, and in challenging the existing problems constructively and optimistically.

Staffing

Staffing patterns need to be more flexible, taking into account the type of illness, degree of dysfunction, and expected recovery. Some areas call for heavier input from physicians; some, additional rehabilitation therapists; and some, increased nursing personnel (those who have bachelor's or master's degrees). Incompetent staff should be replaced, retained, or remotivated. New staff should be obtained at competitive marketplace salaries and benefits for the job so that staff are lured who will stint on neither their time or interest.

Education and Training

Most psychiatric residents in state mental hospitals at present are foreign-born, and their primary need is for acculturation and language instruction. Instead of being used as cheap labor to obviate the need to hire fully licensed physicians, they should receive quality education

and training, especially in such areas as the chronically ill, psychophar-
macology, rehabilitation. In-service training programs for the entire
staff should change from "floor buffing" and form filling to clinical
conferences and didactic presentation of treatment issues. If career
ladders are to remain as methods of advancement, they must be bu-
tressed by genuine educational opportunities provided in the academic
community and by competing mental health teaching services—not
with superficial courses taught by persons with no broader academic or
professional experience than the state hospital.

Physical Structure

The physical plant with which state hospitals are saddled is another area that needs restructuring. Flexible use of the buildings and
grounds would lead to selling some property and renting or buying
space in community settings for treatment activities, changing from a
model of huge monolithic buildings to semimobile modules that could
expand or shrink depending on need, utilization of buildings for rehabilitation activities while moving active treatment functions into the
community, etc. Since closing wards or units does not really save
money—only closing buildings does—there must be pump-priming
monies available if shifts are to be made from institution-based to
community-based locations.

Administrative Structures

Hospitals are still either overcentralized and autocratic or decentralized and inefficient because of a lack of competent clinical and
business administrative staff. This is even more true on a regional or
statewide level. Mental health departments in states like New York are
overstaffed with huge numbers of central or regional office personnel
who, while seemingly busy, in no way contribute to the clinical competence of individual institutions. Somehow private and nonprofit services and hospitals function without this top-heavy bureaucracy—and
much more efficiently than their government counterparts.

A hard look needs to be taken at whether all but a skeleton staff
needs to be retained in the bureaucracy to look after such essential
centralized activities as statistical data-gathering services, communications, and relationships with other state departments. Clinical, administrative and teaching activities should occur at the local level only.
Such a reform of the administrative structure would raise many objec-
tions. It would be fought by centralization-minded bureaucrats, who

do not trust the local facilities' ability to govern themselves and fear loss of their jobs. It would eliminate political interference and the use of the chronic mentally ill as a springboard to career advancement, and it would put an end to the practice of promoting incompetent personnel.

Treatment Programs

Currently, treatment emphasis is on inpatient beds, not total care for the patient-at-risk. A shift to a preventive or Health Maintanence Organization (HMO) approach, a shift rewarding alternatives to hospitalization such as day hospitals or crisis intervention, and a shift from custodial to treatment and activities programs could put the emphasis where it should be—on the needs of the population. As long as the programs encourage the focus on inpatient beds, lengths of inhospital stay, and present staffing rather than responsibility for patient populations and commensurate resources to serve patients, this will be difficult. New funding formulas, reward systems, and professional emphases need to be placed on other than inpatient services.

The Legislature

Legislative reform would include an involvement of legislators and their staffs in the understanding and overseeing of treatment activities for chronic patients. Massive education not only of legislators but also of governmental employees would have to be undertaken to move from the numbers game to quality of care, from attitudes of getting rid of patients who are annoying to the techniques of active treatment and rehabilitation, and from complaining when things do not work to involvement on an ongoing basis.

A system would have to be established where the legislature had competent psychiatric and consumer advice on an ongoing basis, and not as part of the department of mental health's activities. Legislators would have to understand the problem of the lack of a lobby for the severely and chronically mentally ill and weigh this when facing articulate lobbies from other sectors demanding services and/or funding. In addition, an end to the utilization of state hospitals to further political careers would be necessary. Rather than campaigns for superfluous or superficial mental health reforms and finger pointing, a refreshing change would be the candidate's involvement in solving a few of the problems facing the state-funded facility through his charismatic qualities, his community contacts, or his business or legalistic savy.

State Government Agencies'

Departments in the state government would have to become visibly identified when they make decisions controlling clinical care. No longer should state hospitals take the blame for the inability to discharge incompetent or useless employees; the civil service agencies should. No longer should budgetary decisions be faulted to mental healthniks when the bureau of the budget decides on the strictures. And, if the auditing bureau or the office administrating Medicaid, or the department of health imposes new restrictions, policies, and procedures, the public should know who made the decisions and these bureaucrats should be held accountable for the consequences of each decision.

The state departments of mental health also need reforming. In addition to the attitudinal and administrative areas already discussed, there is a desperate need for a clear articulation of the department's goals and objectives, treatment program foci, and clinical concerns. There is not a state department in this country that does not need to devise ways of decreasing the paperwork, increasing the feedback to institutions, representing clinicians and patients to legislators, and becoming an aid to the local hospitals rather than a constraint. Rather than proliferating procedures and policies, a department must function as a central clearing house that fights such proliferation and lobbies for unified accreditation/licensing/control procedures. Instead of issuing new memoranda by the hundreds each week, the central office should give responsibility and resources to the local facility and move into the area of effective and genuine monitoring and accountability. In short, the department should become what a good quarterback or conductor is—a leader, coordinator, articulator and facilitator. It should not attempt to control and direct all areas of activity from afar.

Outside Forces

Attitudes of third-party payors and the public are also in need of attention. It is necessary to educate the general public about the different needs of chronic mental patients, about the effect of overfunding inpatient services rather than providing alternative services, and about the methods of achieving quality psychiatric care, treatment, and rehabilitation. Somehow the wish to get rid of or lock up all persons who are strange, deviant, or different, rather than provide active and effective treatment, must be countered. This does not mean that the solution is freedom to roam about, disturbing others or starving infants; there must be a saner balance between enforced treatment, involving a loss of civil liberties, and freedom to act as one wishes.

The legal profession, too often intent upon suits or actions rather than patients' health, must be educated to a caring point of view. Citizen groups must be formed comprised of concerned constructive individuals who will fight for the fair share of the tax dollar. Unions must represent all their employees, not just the vocal troublemakers. Accrediting and licensing bodies must consolidate their reviews, begin to examine quality not quantity issues, and become a positive not negative force in moving state hospitals into active treatment approaches.

THE PROS OF REFORMING STATE HOSPITALS

In favor of this broad idealistic approach to change all detrimental aspects of state facilities is the fact that this is the system we presently have and it hardly seems sensible to discard it without a conscientious attempt to see if it can function after making the necessary changes. The proposal also retains the principle for which state hospitals were established—to care for those who were not cared for by others, especially the severely and chronically mentally ill. Thus, there is no need to establish a whole new system of mechanism of mental health care delivery if genuine reform can be undertaken.

THE CONS

Many point out that the reforms proposed *are* idealistic and in some cases unrealistic, given the tenor of society and governmental bureaucracies. Such reforms as detailed would be costly, they would go to the heart of entrenched political and professional vested interests, and they would require a long time to become effective. It is also unrealistic to assume that anyone could effectively eliminate the civil service system and political interference and alter public attitudes in the foreseeable future without expending tremendous effort, seizing on or precipitating a crisis, or utilizing exceedingly influential assistance.

CONCLUSIONS

Despite the argument that state hospitals ought to be given a fair chance before they are abandoned, it seems clear that without a total push aimed at remedying all of their deficiencies, they will never succeed. Therefore, partial attempts at redress of the situation probably will lead to the result criticized by true radicals—that of superficial reform and continuing ineffectiveness. The massive investment of money, energy, and time needed to bring about this reform will probably not appeal to enough persons to have it become a vital force. It should be pointed out, however, that this solution is clearly the only one that ensures adequate care for the chronic mental patient as well as improving state hospitals.

REFERENCE

1.   Jones M: Community care for chronic mental patients: The need for a reassessment. Hosp Community Psychiatry 26:94–98, 1975

14

The Pragmatic Solution:
New Roles for
State Hospitals

The proposals to alter the roles and functions of state mental hospitals have increased dramatically in frequency over the past few years. Those that have gained wide acceptance would retain the facilities as such, while altering their now-impossible-to-perform tasks. These proposals would neither require the massive influx of time, money, and energy entailed by the drastic reforms of Chapter 13, nor would they abolish the system. For these reasons the "pragmatic" solutions have great appeal to a large number of politicians and professionals.

THE PROPOSALS

The programatists primarily attack the basic assumption that state hospitals must assume public health responsibility for all persons, with all varieties of mental illness, from all regions of the state. Each proposal divides the mental health "pie" by a different method so that a smaller and more manageable responsibility will be assumed by each individual hospital. The proposals can be grouped under four categories.

Mental health services

1. By geography
2. By patient group (age, diagnosis, chronicity)
3. By specialized function
4. By flexibly fitting state services into the total services mix

Geographic Model

State facilities would no longer serve as all things to all people, as backup facilities to other services in the system, or, more accurately stated, as dumping grounds for the chronic and/or difficult-to-manage patients. A hospital would narrow its sights geographically while widening its services professionally. Thus, it would attempt to become "all things" to a limited number of people. Whether it is formally designated as a community mental health center (CMHC) or not, it might attempt to become one functionally—providing inpatient, outpatient, partial hospitalization, emergency, and crisis services, community consultation and education, etc.[1, 2]

If the hospital narrows its geographic focus, who will assume the remainder of the responsibility? With unified mental health services or community control of state funds and services, such responsibilities can be parceled out, but in states and localities where the systems are discordant, the feasibility of working out such arrangements is less likely.

In favor of this approach is its obvious attempt to get out of the squeeze between both the expectation of responsibility and provision of quality care for a huge number of people and the inadequate resources with which to perform the task. In that it continues the trend on the part of state facilities to move away from custodial care toward active treatment interventions, it will boost morale and attract better qualified professionals to the facility. Those facilities, for instance, in New York State that have higher staff–patient ratios, more active treatment approaches, smaller catchment areas, and newer physical plants —all characteristic of this new CMHC-type state hospital—tend to approach a competitive status with the traditionally higher status institutions.

In older hospitals, however, with decrepit buildings, entrenched staff members, and a traditional custodial orientation the situation is different. A community faced with a choice of being served totally by this traditional state hospital versus a more active treatment facility will react predictably. The inequality of staff competence, salaries and benefits, training and research and quality of treatment and care offered by the older state hospital compared to that offered by CMHCs, nonprofit hospitals, and private facilities will pose sizable problems for mental health planners and administrators seeking to work out rearrangements in geographic responsibility. There will also be problems for the consumers affected and their elected representatives.

Patient Groups

Proposals that use patient groups as the basis for their operations would have state facilities assume responsibility not for all persons in a limited geographic area, but for a limited number of certain types of patients in a wider area. Thus, since most CMHCs and nonprofit hospitals have active emergency services, outpatient clinics and short-term inpatient wards, they would assume the care of patients needing these services. State facilities, on the other hand, would then be freer to concentrate on other patient groups. Admittedly, to date this has meant custodial care for the chronic mental patients whom no one else wishes to treat, but the advocates of this approach are hopeful that active treatment, care, and rehabilitation services would be developed to cope with the chronic mental patient—and that the result would not be simply a repetition of custodial care. The patients targeted for such a division of patient responsibility include adult chronic mental patients,[3-6] children and youth,[3, 5, 7] the elderly,[3, 5] abusers of alcohol and drugs,[3, 5] the chronically ill, (medical and mental),[8] criminal offenders,[3] the mentally retarded,[5] and the mentally disturbed blind, deaf, and multiply handicapped.

The attractive features of this sort of division of labor include its generally agreed-upon assumption of responsibility for care and treatment of the chronically mentally ill and the attempt to stop the competition between all mental health services for the small pool of patients. The responsibility would be divided.

There are several obvious deficiencies. Grouping may lead once again to custodial, second-class treatment of those patients seen as unappealing or untreatable. It retains the same staff, staffing, patients, buildings, bureaucracy, etc., of the state hospital system, and it places the state facility back into a role it has been trying to avoid for the past two decades—that of treater of last resort and fill-in of gaps in services by default.

Specialized Functions

The division of responsibility is not by patient category but by specialized function. Here the division of labor makes for more diversity and the blurring of patient types. It also conceptualizes the functions provided by state facilities versus other mental health services in a new way. If we use the model prevalent in health planning currently as the one projected for the future, the state facilities would offer teritiary care services, backing up the primary and secondary care services in the communities.

Functions that have been suggested as appropriate for state facilities to assume include long-term care,[4, 9] residential care,[3] research,[4] teaching,[4] care for patients who need separation from their families and the environment,[4] forensic services including evaluation,[5] and rehabilitation of chronic or crisis-prone individuals.[10] Rosen argues effectively that the sort of care provided by some state facilities in terms of rehabilitation services for the long-term patient, including quarterway and halfway houses, Fairweather lodges, day hospitals and therapeutic workshops, are uniquely suited to state hospitals and will be lost if such facilities are not maintained.[10]

This division of responsibility does ensure care for those who might not otherwise receive it—e.g., care for long-term patients, which is discriminated against by all private and governmental third-party reimbursers. It provides centralized services that are too expensive for any single catchment area to fund (e.g., forensic services), and it designates certain functions as uniquely the province of state facilities rather than forcing second-class services on them.

Against the proposal is the fact that once again it does not attempt to alter the institution, its staff, staffing, buildings, etc., but merely its job. In addition, while the functions designated may be seen by some to be unique, they may also be perceived once again as second-class and second-rate.

Flexibility in Functioning

The last method of "slicing the pie" is the most creative and potentially different. It calls upon state facilities to assume a different role in every catchment area, fitting into the area's existing range of services, providing whatever services are needed, addressing whatever needs are not being met, and serving whatever patient groups are not being served. The model is really a combination of the first three proposals, taking into consideration the particular network of services in a community.

Alternative proposals suggest that the state hospital fit into the mental health network,[9, 11, 12] the total health network,[13] or the human services network.[14] Regardless of which network the state hospitals fit into, however, most experts agree that they must either creatively interlock with other services or face obsolescence if the hospital is not flexible enough to alter its role to meet changing needs.

There are several worthy features of this proposal. It is an adaptive position for state hospitals, ensuring their survival by filling realistic identified needs in the mental health network. But, as with the prior proposals, it leaves the state hospital system as it is, a situation that may breed further scandals and problems in time. In addition, the assumption that each state facility is flexible enough to respond to the changing and unique needs of a particular area is an assumption that may not be warranted, and the vested interests within the facility may cause such a proposal to go awry.

OTHER PROPOSALS

There are two other proposals which deserve mention and both relate more to the way state hospitals are funded than to their roles. The first provides for a new state facility, that is a state-funded service with new buildings, a comprehensive mandate, fuller funding for more complete staffing, and a smaller geographical responsibility. An example of this is the Illinois zone center, which while state-funded, cannot be classified as a traditional state hospital.[2] Proponents of this model argue that it proves that facilities that are state-funded and state-run, are not necessarily second-class.

The other idea, proposed by Eaton,[13] suggests that state hospitals will function in the future as nonprofit corporations with prepayment arrangements. Such funding would certainly free them of many of the governmental constraints mentioned previously as well as provide incentives for more innovative treatment programming, which is not encouraged by current funding arrangements.

THE PROS FOR CHANGING HOSPITAL ROLES

Three points can be made in favor of changing the roles of the state hospitals. Foremost, it does not scrap the system. In addition, the property, jobs, and programs managed by the states are preserved, and it is a cheaper alternative than total reform of the system.

THE CONS

The principal argument against the success of these proposals to alter the roles of the state mental hospitals is that while they preserve the system, they preserve it relatively unchanged and thus offer no better solution to the current mess than a different role. In addition, unless there are drastic changes in state employee unions, civil service regulations, salaries and benefits, etc., there will not be parity within the entire network of mental health services. And this can lead to considerable difficulty. There is little assurance that a second-class system will not result, a system like the present one where scandals will continue to occur and patients continue to be underserved.

CONCLUSIONS

The options discussed in this chapter most probably will be selected by most states to improve their mental health delivery services since they are inexpensive, preserve the existing system, and do not disturb the status quo. The test will be whether patient care in the state hospitals or all of the mental health system improves. Merely holding on to the political, bureaucratic, and vested interests of the state mental hospitals is not enough. If care and treatment of the severely and chronically mentally ill does not improve, if a revision of roles merely perpetuates a 2-class system, and if redivision of the mental health pie becomes another administrative maneuver rather than clinical advancement, those options will not have long-term value and further reform or change will be necessary.

REFERENCES

1. Bonn E, Binner PR, Huber HM: Evolution of a modern state hospital: The Fort Logan Mental Health Center experience, in Zusman J, Bertsch EF (eds): The Future Role of the State Hospital. Lexington, Mass. Lexington Books, 1975
2. DeVito RA, Tapley R: A View into a Modern State Hospital Operated Mental Health Facility. Springfield, Ill., Thomas, 1975
3. Demone HW, Schulberg HC: Has the state mental hospital a future as a human service resource? in Zusman J, Bertsch EF (eds): The Future Role of the State Hospital. Lexington, Mass, Lexington Books, 1975
4. Stewart DW: The future of the state mental hospital. Perspec Psychiatr Care 13:120–122, 1975
5. Horizon House Institute: The Future Role of State Mental Hospital: A National Survey of Planning and Program Trends. Philadelphia, the Author, 1975

6. Lamb HR, Goertzel V: The demise of the state mental hospital—premature obituary: Arch Gen Psychiatry 26:489–495, 1972
7. Institutionalization: An Editorial. Newsletter, Society for Adolescent Psychiatry, Summer 1973
8. Action for Mental Health: The Final Report of the Joint Commission on Mental Illness and Health. New York, Basic Books, 1961
9. Ozarin LD, Levenson AI: The future of the public mental hospital. Am J Psychiatry 125:1647–1652, 1969
10. Rosen IM: In further defense of the state hospital: Its rehabilitative function. Hosp Community Psychiatry 27:820–821, 1976
11. Greenblatt M: The public psychiatric hospital: Room for optimism. Am J Psychiatry 127:1397–1398, 1971
12. Talbott JA: Developments in metropolitan state hospital services, in Zusman J, Bertsch EF (eds): The Future Role of the State Hospital. Lexington, Mass., Lexington Books, 1975
13. Eaton MT: The future of the public mental hospital, in Arieti S (ed): American Handbook of Psychiatry (vol 6). New York, Basic Books, 1975
14. Higashi W: The hospital's role in the delivery of services. Unpublished paper

15
The Radical Solution:
Closing State Hospitals

The proposal to scrap the state hospital system is not new. Since there is little evidence that state facilities have performed their tasks sufficiently well in the past 100 years to merit their continuing existence, demand for their aboliton has been voiced periodically, and increasingly so during the past 20 years. Solomon, in his presidential address at the American Psychiatric Association Annual Meeting in 1958, called for an end to state hospitals.[1] The Joint Commission on Mental Health and Illness, which reportedly initially favored this position, recommended in 1961 that no more large state hospitals be built and that they be replaced, in large part, by a network of community-based outpatient clinics.[2]

After the Canadian province of Saskatchewan in the 1960s decided to phase out mental hospitals, several states in this country planned similar moves,[3] but the problems encountered in the 1970s, most notably in Massachusetts, California, and New York, put a damper on this solution.[4] Not only were communities up in arms over the de-institutionalization process, which dumped thousands of ex-mental patients into neighborhoods that then became ghettos of the mentally ill, but also other segments of the public were opposed. Unions, fearing an end to thousands of jobs, businessmen in communities housing large state hospitals, facing major losses in their businesses, and elected representatives, faced with opposition from all sides, all began to exert pressure to force the states to step back from the closure solution. By 1975 a survey revealed that only 5 states of 44 responding intended further closures of state hospitals.[5] Today there are still some who call for this solution, believing that we are better off without *any* mental hospitals.[6]

THE PROPOSAL

The proposal put forth by the proponents of closure is a simple one. Basically, it provides for the closing of state mental hospitals through a combination of consolidation of facility populations, discharge of patients into the community, and picking up of persons in need of treatment by nonstate, community-based mental health services.

In some states the plan, while never articulated, was formulated during the reduction in state hospital populations under de-institutionalization. It seemed logical that the decrease would proceed to the point where no patients would be hospitalized and the hospital could then close. Other states planned for a transfer of patients to another hospital once a core number in each facility was reached. The staff of the sending hospital would be retrained for community services, and the facility closed. Other states made definite plans for increasing local government resources and facilities to care for the de-institutionalized population, thinking that with increasing community ability to care for patients the need for state services would diminish, and eventually disappear.

THE PROBLEMS

There were three problems with the way closure was attempted in the 1970s in most states. First, the anticipated opposition by a coalition of union and community forces in most instances was answered by governmental rhetoric instead of by adequate preparation, retraining of employees, and establishment of quality community care facilities.[7] Second, there was no provision for a full range of services to care for these severely and chronically mentally ill individuals in the community.[8] Third, the debate continues as to whether chronic mental patients can ever be properly handled by other-than-state facilities, given the nature and needs of their illness.[9,10] If closure is ever to succeed there must be (1) adequate preparation and retraining of state employees, (2) adequate and comprehensive quality services in the community, funded at adequate levels, and (3) specific provisions made for care, treatment, and rehabilitation of the chronic mental patient.

THE PROS FOR CLOSURE

In favor of the proposal to close state mental hospitals is the promise that we will finally be rid of a system that seems never to have done its job to anyone's satisfaction. Second, it may save money, despite the need to pump a great deal of money initially into the community facilities and despite the money drain occasioned by two systems (state and community) overlapping for a period of time. Third, it moves patient care into the twentieth century, where active intervention, optimistic rehabilitation, and treatment near family and friends will be optimal.

THE CONS

The arguments by the opponents to closure are numerous: It will be very difficult to convince the taxpayer and legislator that two systems need to be equally well funded *before* the older one can be phased out. Community facilities may indeed continue to be unwilling to care for the most severely and chronically mentally ill and prefer the retention of a backup custodial care asylum somewhere. Businesses and state employees will suffer since they will not be able to adapt to the shift in locus of services and patients. Dislocation of patients is antitherapeutic and, in fact, morbidity- and mortality-inducing. Having failed the first time around, it will fail again.

CONCLUSIONS

While closure seemed to present the ideal solution in the 1950s, the backlash against it and the failure to provide adequate and effective community alternatives to state mental hospitals have probably doomed its viability as an option at this point. On the other hand, increasing economic pressures and continuing state hospital scandals may precipitate its readoption. Since it is not likely that adequate community support systems will then be provided, the scandalous conditions that originally occurred at the height of de-institutionalization will reappear in the community.

REFERENCES

1. Solomon H: Presidential address 1958. Am J Psychiatry 115:1–9, 1958
2. Action for Mental Health: The Final Report of the Joint Commission on Mental Illness and Health. New York, Basic Books, 1961
3. Stewart A, LaFave HG, Grunberg F, Herjanic M: Problems in phasing out a large public mental hospital. Am J Psychiatry 125:82–88, 1968
4. Where is my home?: The closing of state mental hospitals. Hosp Community Psychiatry 25:393–401, 1974
5. Horizon House Institute: The Future Role of State Mental Hospitals: A National Survey of Planning and Program Trends. Philadelphia, the Author, 1975
6. Mendel WM: On the abolition of the psychiatric hospital, in Roberts LM, Greenfield NS, Miller MH (eds): Comprehensive Mental Health. Madison, University of Wisconsin Press, 1968
7. Greenblatt M. Galzier E: The phasing out of mental hospitals in the United States. Am J Psychiatry 132:1135–1140, 1975
8. Becker A, Schulberg HC: Phasing out state hospitals—A psychiatric dilemma. N Eng J Med 294:255–261, 1976
9. Jones M: As cited in The changing mental hospital: Emerging alternatives. Hosp Community Psychiatry 25:386–392, 1974
10. Lamb HR, Goertzel V: The demise of the state hospital—a premature obituary? Arch Gen Psychiatry 26:489–495, 1972

PART V

Reality and the Future

16
Guidelines, Not Solutions

The final answer to the problems posed by and encountered by state mental hospitals may not be arrived at by consideration of whether they should be closed, kept, or modified—but rather by consideration of what the needs are and trying to address those needs through a fresh problem-solving effort. If we begin by addressing the need to provide treatment, care, and rehabilitation for the severely and chronically mentally ill, including certain special populations (e.g., the aged, criminal offenders, etc.), it may well be that although we need to have active treatment programs, adequate community care programs, abundant rehabilitation facilities, and high-quality asylums, they do not necessarily need to be state-funded and state-run. Indeed, while some new state facilities, such as the Illinois zone centers, have been extemely successful, the care of the severely and chronically mentally ill can probably be provided much better by non state facilities.

If we take into consideration our collective responsibility for both the vulnerable chronic-prone population involved and the residual system of state mental hospitals, none of the four solutions proposed in Part IV is ideal. Both the conservative (keeping state hospitals) and pragmatic (modifying their role) solutions, while utilizing the existing system, do nothing to change the factors that lead to low-quality care, bureaucratic nightmares, and media scandals. The radical solution (closure) does, but at the price of scrapping the system and with no guarantee that the severely and chronically ill will be well served. The only solution that carries both the promise of improving the basic problems of the state hospital as well as caring for chronic mental patients is that of a drastic and wide-sweeping reform—a solution that, while appealing, is so utopian as to be impractical for serious consideration given the political and bureaucratic forces at present.

Instead of looking to these four solutions, we are better off spelling out guidelines that should underlie any approach in improving the lot of the state hospital and the lot of the chronic mental patient, if these efforts are to be successful.

THE PRIMARY FOCUS MUST BE THE PATIENT

We must begin by focusing primarily on the chronic mental patient and his or her needs. Thus, we must *not* begin by concentrating on the system's needs (e.g., retention of jobs, status, etc.), or on the economic problems of various levels of government, or on the politician's problem of selling whatever programs are proposed—although later these must be considered in the process of implementing whatever plan can best provide for these patients.

First, chronic mental patients need a range of graded services that progress from inpatient facilities (with both active treatment and asylum elements) to community care programs. These services include a variety of increasingly independent treatment settings *as well as* a range of graded living situations that may or may not correlate exactly with the treatment settings. Figure 16–1 demonstrates both the spectrum of necessary treatment services as well as the spectrum of needed living situations. Optionally, treatment opportunities must range from pre-hospital services (e.g., crisis intervention) through inpatient services, to aftercare and rehabilitation services. Likewise, living settings must vary from prehospital (e.g., partial hospital) through inpatient, to independent living arrangements.

Second, a method must be found by which the intricate and contradictory rules and regulations involving funding for chronic mental patients can be made more rational so that financial support for the patient's treatment *and* housing arrangements is provided no matter where the patient is. We should no longer allow Medicaid to fund some governmental hospitals (e.g., county and city) and not others (e.g., state), or provide excellent expensive inpatient treatment but inadequate and cheap home care, or support rehabilitation for patients who demonstrate positive progress but not for those who would return to state hospitals without it.

Third, we must find a way to change the existing reimbursement

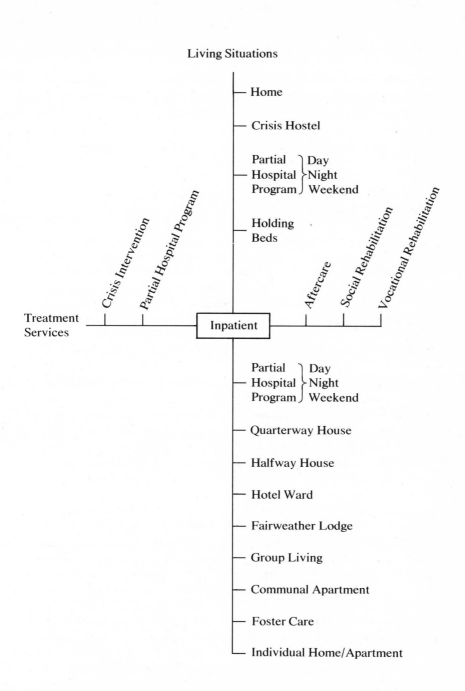

Fig. 16–1. The spectrum of optimal treatment services and living situations.

mechanisms that reward full beds and inpatient services and penalize empty beds and outpatient services. It has been known for at least a half a century that our dependence on expensive hospital services runs counter to both good treatment practices and economic prudence. If outpatient care were reimbursed at six times the level of inpatient care —a reversal of the present situation—care patterns would change immediately and drastically.

A SHIFT IN THINKING ABOUT THE CHRONIC AND CHRONIC-PRONE PATIENT

In addition to beginning by focusing on the patient rather than on the health care system, we must revise our awareness of, attitudes about, and status of concepts concerning the care and treatment of the persons who are or become chronic mental patients. The general public, our elected representatives, patients, and professionals must all appreciate that chronic mental patients are different in several important ways from others suffering from mental illness.

They are in need of long-term care and treatment as well as long-term living arrangements. Their treatment and everyday requirements (e.g., housing, clothing, food) will necessitate concern and funding for a lifetime in most instances. The goal of any involvement with this population is not cure but care, and there must be a system to track such individuals, since they are so prone to fall between the cracks or become extruded from society, social subsystems, and health care networks or services. Their care needs to be coordinated by someone since they cannot negotiate and manage their own problem solving. Along with this, a designation of who is responsible for their treatment, care, and rehabilitation must be made—instead of the current system of chance, fragmentation and uncoordination. Lastly, the disparate elements of the mental health, health, and social systems must cooperate effectively to better serve this population and cease adhering to their own idiosyncratic guidelines and special target populations.

Overriding these goals is the urgent need for all of us to understand that chronic mental patients cannot speak up or lobby for themselves and need others to be their advocates. Legislators and the broader society need to decide on how much investment they are willing to put into this group and state it publicly.

AN IMPROVED CHANGE PROCESS

There must be a different and better process of implementing changes in the delivery of mental health services. There should be a clearly stated and understood mandate for change, if such is desired, from elected officials, the legislative groups responsible for such areas, and the governmental departments involved with mental health. The objectives of mental health programs, especially when they involve change, must be clearly thought out, fully understood, and clearly articulated. There must be visibility and accessibility of decision makers and the decision process. There must be support by the citizens whose taxes will fund mental health programs, as well as the citizens who will receive such services, as to the initiation, change, or maintenance of such programs. There must be active, strong, effective leadership and an adequate number of active patient-oriented persons who will implement new or changing programs. Lastly, there must be increased attention paid to weeding out those persons in the system who, for personal, professional, or institutional reasons, constitute destructive influences, harbor inappropriate mentalities, or possess potentialities for resistance.

MAJOR SHIFTS IN THINKING ABOUT FUNDING

Concommitant changes are necessary in the way governmental and private insurance authorities view funding of services for serious mental illness. These include new funding formulas, new modes of funding, the separation of funding *for* and provision *of* services, and redistribution of funding.

Funding formulae must be revised so as not to reward institutionalization and dependence (e.g., inpatient care) and penalize ambulatory services. They must also make provision for the chronicity of mental illness through mechanisms to ensure ongoing long-term treatment, with the understanding that some funding is for terminal placement, maintenance treatment, and stabilizing care situations. Money has to follow patients, especially if further shifts in their locus are contemplated. For example, funds must leave institutions along with patients going into community settings and be used for these settings. It is necessary to devise more flexible methods of funding and moving money within budgets if patients rather than programs are to be served.

Rather than running so many mental health services itself, the government should utilize new methods of funding services and patients to allow for patients to select their care facility and to reward preventive and ambulatory services rather than inpatient beds. Certainly if a form of national health insurance is enacted by Congress that allows for equal, nondiscriminatory reimbursement for *all* mental health services, it will produce dramatic changes in consumer utilization patterns. A voucher system, proposed by some for educational and housing services, that allows every American to choose where he or she wants treatment, even at differing rates but with equivalent total dollar amounts in vouchers, would also engender marked shifts in utilization. Health Maintenance Organizations (HMOs) that provide total services for a population and where utilization of ambulatory services decreases the need for and cost of inpatient services is another promising approach. And lastly, government should make more ample use of contracts for services, allowing private and nonprofit hospitals to bid against government-run hospitals. These institutions, because of their relative lack of bureaucracy and administrative constraints, may be able to deliver more services, at a lower cost, to the patient and taxpayer.

Such contracting out of services by government would not only hold the promise of a higher quality, lower cost service, but also get government out of the business of the direct provision of mental health services and move it into quality control, contracts and monitoring, and planning and forecasting for entire populations. Services could then be coordinated locally and not run by a central government agency, which, as we have seen, has a poor record for such.

It is clear to many in the field of mental health that there is enough money to provide quality services in many areas. The problems are not the quantity of the services and the total amount of money available for them but the quality of the services and the distribution of the funds. More and more of the taxpayers' dollar goes into maintenance of the bureaucracy at the expense of patient care. New record forms, devised by the hundreds of governmental and private agencies that oversee and regulate hospitals, swamp service providers, and staff must take time from essential duties to complete them. State and county departments of mental health are bloated with technocrats who offer no assistance with what should be the object of such systems— patient care. The elimination of sizable portions of the centralized bureaucracies that both administer and operate governmental mental health services would go a long way toward redistributing the money spent. If government agencies were divested of the conflict-of-interest situation they now find themselves in, that of running and funding services, they could devote their time to devising strategies to make programs fit patients' needs rather than force patients into programs that are government-operated, in order to perpetuate these programs. The proposal to strip government of its own services will be difficult to implement unless there is strong support from the highest levels and involves key political decision makers. Until it is done, however, we will continue to have a situation where there is probably enough money in the entire system, but it is so misspent and misallocated that it cannot be brought to bear upon the problems of patient care.

NEW FORMS OF RESPONSIBILITY AND ACCOUNTABILITY

If resources are allocated according to patient needs rather than vested interests, a step will be taken toward giving someone or an institution the responsibility and commensurate resources for doing a task and then being accountable for the performance. Thus, we would move toward a new accountability—one in which the person or institution could be held accountable because they have been given sufficient resources and tools to accomplish the tasks they were given the authority and responsibility to do.

This new accountability, however, must not be managed in the traditional manner, which is perfunctory paperwork accountability by government, until political or media accountability forces scandalous conditions out into the open. Rather, the public must have a running account of what is being done, so that quality patient care rather than electioneering so selling newspapers becomes the drive behind public interest. It is difficult to reward excellence rather than scandal, and to date we have been unable to devise methods of doing this because scandal not excellence wins campaigns and sells newspapers. But the challenge should be met.

NEW ATTITUDES FOR LEADERSHIP

Leadership in mental health services must be placed in the hands of those who value people and quality and taken away from those who thrive on paper and quantity. As I have demonstrated repeatedly in previous chapters, attention to paperwork, regulations, and form filling, is an active defense against grappling with the frustrations of treating the severely and chronically mentally ill. If we are to move in any direction but a continuing downward spiral, we must put a halt to the utilization of this avoidance maneuver and return to leaders who value people, patients, and programs.

In addition, the leadership of mental health services must focus on eliminating constraints and restrictions and begin to facilitate quality patient care. The reward system should provide incentives for quality and against quantity. National health insurance holds promise of assisting this development if it engenders decentralization and freedom of choice by patients—but it promises only nightmares if it introduces a new centralized bureaucracy with hundreds of new constraints and forms.

A PUBLIC CONSTITUENCY FOR THE SEVERELY AND CHRONICALLY MENTALLY ILL

Throughout the history of attempts by American society to deal with chronic mental patients run the threads of an inability to provide quality services for this population, resulting in a dependence on mediocre governmental services. Except for the providers of mental health services, who are always correctly perceived as not disinterested observers, there has been no effective public constituency for the severely and chronically mentally ill. While such a constituency may never develop from the patients and families of the severely ill, it can develop from concerned citizens and neighbors. Although destructive in many ways, de-institutionalization may have started this process. Neither I, nor anyone I know, understands how this constituency will develop, but without it the fate of the most neglected of society's children will continue to be in the hands of politicians and the press rather than the citizenry.

WHAT THE RESULTING SYSTEM MIGHT LOOK LIKE

Taking the premise stated at the start of this chapter, that we should begin with the problems as they exist and then devise new solutions, we can look at two major issues—the needs of the severely and chronically mentally ill and the work of the mental health system to care for this population. The needs of the patients are many, but certainly they include, as has been repeatedly stressed in this volume, continuity of care, permanent funding, and a range of coordinated and graded treatment services and living situations. The work of the system is to provide quality care and treatment, and to provide it both effectively (concentrating on outcome) and efficiently (diminishing bureaucratic defenses).

It is clear to me that the way to attain these objectives is through a unified mental health system with regional rather than central control— a system that would not run services but contract for them, that would have provisions for patients to buy their own care (through vouchers or national health insurance) that would provide tracking of patients wherever they are, and that would regard state facilities as only one institution among a number of institutions rather than *the one* to be protected. In some areas of the country such a system would readily result in patients electing to abandon former state and county hospitals for private and nonprofit facilities. The state mental hospital might well close as a result of this redistribution of patients and resultant services. On the other hand, in areas where there are few other choices, state facilities might continue to serve as the asylum component in a comprehensive network of graded services for the severely and chronically mentally ill.

It is a common observation that in terms of governmental politics and efficiency state departments are better run than county or city ones and federal departments better run than state ones. On the other hand, we also know that the provision of clinical services is best done on the lowest level possible. Thus, ideally, funding and regulation would be at the federal level, and provision of services at the local level. A model for this is the Medicare program, which certainly functions better than Medicaid, state mental health services, or county hospitals. However, there is a huge gap between federal authority and local patient care, and this would probably best be filled by a catchment-area "czar," preferably the largest provider in an area, whose responsibility it would be to coordinate all mental health services in an area. Such a system, gets government out of its conflict-of-interest position of both funding and running mental health services and puts it in a position of contracting with local providers and monitoring their provision of services. With this system we would have the elimination of a huge inefficient bureaucracy, the clear designation of responsibility with adequate resources to providers of service to the severely and chronically mentally ill, and the hope for finally applying the tools of modern active treatment, care and rehabilitation to this needful population.

17

Major Themes and Portents of the Future

This chapter will touch briefly on each of the important points raised, discuss several of the underlying major themes, and then consider several broader theoretical issues that this study has illustrated. It will conclude with some predictions of the future of state hospitals, governmental psychiatry, and psychiatry.

MAJOR ISSUES

Why Study State Hospitals

It is important to examine state mental hospitals for several reasons. First, they represent a major component, albeit diminishing, of services in our mental health system. At one time they were almost the sole provider of services in this country. Although they now provide less than one-tenth of the total services, they continue to use approximately 22 percent of the monies spent for mental health services and 80 percent of state mental health budgets, which themselves are often second in size only to education budgets.

Second, despite numerous attempts at reform, innovation, and modification, the hospital system still does not do a good job. Recently, with the advent of de-institutionalization, it has become more obvious how difficult it is to treat and care for the chronically mentally ill. The study of the failure of an institution specifically designed to handle this problem should provide some insight to our future attempts to care for this population.

Third, state mental hospitals represent a long-standing attempt on the part of government to provide direct medical services. As such, they represent a prime example of government medicine, an area of possible expansion in the near future.

Fourth, the state hospital system demonstrates both the positive and negative aspects of the effects of a bureaucratic structure on human service problems. As government assumes more and more responsibility for human services, it may be wise to reexamine whether or not the bureaucratic model fits these tasks as well as other nonhuman services.

Fifth, with the imminent arrival of a governmental program of national health insurance there will be shifts in the patterns of utilization of facilities and services. It is important to predict the impact of this new funding force on a major component of the health care field.

Sixth, the process of reform and change in state hospitals is a fascinating one. A great deal has happened in the century-plus of their existence, and there is much to be learned about the differences between cosmetic and substantive change through a study of this social institution.

Lastly, the state mental hospitals demonstrate, perhaps better than any other system, how a social institution reacts to both problems in performing its task and in handling threats from the outside world by adapting and responding in such a way as to defend itself rather than address the root (radical) causes of its difficulties. This process, seen in a system, is so akin to that observed in the defensive structure of individuals that "sick systems" could conceivably benefit from "analysis" and "treatment" in much the same manner as sick individuals do.

What Can Be Learned from the History of State Hospitals

The first thing that strikes us about the historical development of state mental hospitals is that they, along with other social institutions, have failed to address successfully the most pressing problem facing them and for which they were created—the care, treatment, and rehabilitation of the severely and chronically mentally ill. Psychiatry continues to be frustrated by the elusiveness and intractability of this severely vulnerable and impaired population, and it is certainly time to examine the reasons for this situation.

In addition, we have learned that shifting the locus of care and funding of the mentally ill from families to county almshouses, to state mental hospitals, to federally funded community mental health centers has done little more than complicate the delivery of mental health services and facilitate buck-passing, promote neglect of the difficult to threat, and encourage various levels of government to shift blame, responsibility, and economic liability.

We have seen that the pendulum, which from the time of colonial America to sometime after World War II swung from local to centralized care of the mentally ill, has since World War II swung back toward decentralization, both in the entire mental health system and its subsystems (e.g., state hospitals). This shift from decentralization to centralization, back to decentralization, which is not unique to mental health, has revealed some of the strengths and weaknesses of both polar extremes.

Recent history has brought to the fore a most perplexing dilemma —that of the quality of life for the severely impaired mental patient. As a progressive, liberal, democratic society, we have been particularly preoccupied in recent years with a myriad of individual and human rights. In the shift of the severely and chronically mentally ill from state institutions to nursing homes and "community" welfare hotels and flophouses we have had to wrestle with the dilemma concerning where patients are better off and how important is the quality of their life in comparison with their level of functioning, individual wishes, and necessity for treatment.

An analysis of historical developments has also illustrated some of the economic issues pertaining to the treatment of the mentally ill. Funding controls the quality, quantity, and locus of treatment, and more and more decisions that might better be made by a clinical problem-solving process are determined by financial pressures. Government is in a profound conflict-of-interest position. On the one hand, it operates its own mental health services, and on the other hand, it funds private and non-profit services—controlling the spigots for both with an admittedly not unbiased hand.

Our historical review of state hospitals has demonstrated that a serious problem in adequately funding quality mental health services relates to the lack of a constituency for mental health services to compete actively with other citizens for a fair share of the tax dollar. In the absence of such a grass-roots interest both funding and policy decisions are left to governmental bodies, which as just mentioned, are not disinterested observers.

Getting a Grasp on the Problems of State Hospitals

To grasp the complexity of the problems posed by and faced by state mental hospitals, one must look at them from several angles: their constraints in operating, the political bath they are immersed in, the attitudes of the people who work for and have authority over them, and the elements in their organizational structure.

The number of "givens" (those stolid, seemingly immutable factors that predetermine so much of what does and will happen) that state hospitals must live with seems extraordinary. Whether we are talking about patients, programs, administrative procedures, buildings, or governmental processes, we are struck by the limitation on the degrees of freedom that hospitals have. Most oppressive are probably those of the patient population (the severely and chronically mentally ill) and the administrative structure (the governmental bureaucracy). It is probably because of these incredible number of constraints and strictures that most persons frustrated with state mental hospitals have the impulse to scrap the system. To try to change or even budge the hundreds of little rules, regulations, and procedural obstacles just a bit seems so futile.

In addition, the problems of the system are compounded by its place in the political process. It has no power base. To operate effectively in any political game, the players must have some power chits. In state mental hospitals neither the care receivers nor care providers have such tokens.

Another major problem facing state hospitals is an attitudinal one. The attitudes of all participants in the situation seem destined to undermine its effectiveness. The average citizen's fear and wish to have the "crazies" put away, the civil servant's wish to survive the next day and put in 20 years, and the care giver's desire to avoid the frustration of dealing with difficult patients all work against the goal of quality care for the patient.

Many of the problems encountered can be seen as part of a defensive structure erected to avoid the frustration of dealing with difficult patients. It seems clear that this is a primary area for potential change. Paperwork, attention to statistics, power struggles, and "Mickey-Mouse" rules and regulations all have become weapons in the war against dealing with patients and are major factors in the hospitals' failure to perform their purpose—the care and treatment of their patients. The way the system has established priorities, rewards, and punishments, and the administrative procedures followed, also seem to predict further failure. When bed censuses and cleanliness are rewarded rather than quality of care and program effectiveness, it is clear what the outcome will be. Likewise, when responsibility and accountability are not commensurate with resources and authority, the result is equally preordained. The system encourages not clinical care, but administrative detail, and to the outsider it seems designed to fail.

The Change Process in State Hospital

A fascinating dilemma confronts us on examination of the process of change in state institutions. While scandals have been uncovered since the initiation of the state hospital system, few substantive changes for the better have been effected, in contrast with numerous cosmetic repairs. Why is it that change seems so difficult to attempt in state hospitals?

As stated earlier, it is probably because there are so many obstacles that have been set up, intentionally or unintentionally, that to knock each one down is just too time-consuming a process. The attempt to change state facilities has been so frustrating that it constitutes another reason behind the impulse to scrap them altogether.

Despite the lack of progress in change efforts, however, much can be learned about the change process itself from the state hospitals' attempts to change. We know that multiple tactics are needed, that there are several key prerequisites to successful change, and that change processes may be quite different in different systems. Our analysis of the change process has also thrown some light on the lives of change agents—how they operate, react to frustration, and adapt or do not adapt to the system. We have seen that a crucial understanding of the processes underlying institutional stability can come from an understanding of the resistances encountered in the change process.

Probably the most promising approach to examine, if we hope to change the care of the severely and chronically mentally ill, is that of altering the entire mental health system. Approaches that involve only subsystems or compartmentalized elements in a system may produce certain felicitous results, but they will not affect the more deeply implanted problems. It is only by an overall systems approach that we may see genuine promise for change, both in mental health and in other areas.

What the Search for Solutions Proves

In examining the possible solutions to the problems faced by state hospitals, several observations can be made. It becomes even more obvious than before that many of the problems which are present represent defenses against dealing with difficult patients. The push to retain state hospitals or modify them slightly but not implement drastic change seems designed to retain the system, save jobs, preserve people's status in the mental health field, etc. rather than find the best solution for the severely and chronically mentally ill.

The examination of possible proposed solutions brings out the problem that government has in defending its bureaucracy and territory. Governmental bodies, in this instance, no longer attempt to help their constituents and local agencies solve problems but spend inordinate time and money on protecting what they have.

It also becomes apparent that total and sweeping reform is a very expensive procedure and that given the inclination of government and the frustration of the policymakers and care givers, there is a great temptation once again to attempt only some narrow changes in the roles of state facilities. The issue of cosmetic change is one that must become apparent to the public and legislators at some point. When it does, and if they exercise their power, this mechanism may no longer be an option.

It also appears obvious from this study that the impulse to scrap the state hospital system is still present. Despite its failure the first time, the continuing economic crunch and the continuing frustration of mental health professionals and administrators may push this option into consideration again. If a new phase-out attempt is made in an unprepared, precipitous, and money-saving manner, it will again create many more new problems that would have to be dealt with than it will solve.

SUMMARY OF IMPORTANT THEMES

State Hospitals Have Failed in Their Mission

State hospitals were established to care for the severely and chronically mentally ill in a safe, humane manner because communities and local facilities were unable to do so. Since their founding the hospitals have been attacked as inhumane, substandard, understaffed, and providing only poor custodial care. Attempts to change the situation have tended to be either cosmetic or to involve narrowing of their broad tasks.

Resources Must Match Responsibilities

A major reason that state hospitals have failed is that they have never been given adequate resources and commensurate authority to fulfill their responsibility, for which they can be held accountable. This failure is the fault of the public, its elected officials, the mental health professions, and governmental departments of mental health. Each and every one has failed to articulate and publicize the actual needs, costs, and consequences of inadequate tools and resources so that even if a decision is made not to provide adequate resources, the public, patients and care providers clearly understand this inequity.

Chronic Mental Patients Are Difficult To Treat

A root problem in the failure of state hospitals is the difficult nature of their primary population—the severely and chronically mentally ill. Serious mental illness may sometimes be contained and patients maintained through aggressive follow-up, a multiplicity of treatment interventions, and continuing psychopharmacological therapy. In most cases, though, in addition, there will always be a need not only for repeated rehospitalization and crisis intervention, but also for attention to primary needs (housing, income, activity, food) as well as social and vocational habilitation and rehabilitation. This constitutes a massive therapeutic/social effort with meticulous attention to detail and completeness in a population that neither expresses its appreciation for such heroic efforts nor responds to provide the care givers with intrinsic satisfaction for their attempts.

Moving the Locus of Care Does Not Solve the Problems

A traditional approach to the problem of caring for the chronic mental patient is to shift the locus of care and level of funding (family→county→state→federal→community, etc.). This does not solve the problem. It merely aggravates it by creating a huge patchwork system, or more correctly nonsystem, of mental health services. Just as care givers out of frustration with dealing with chronic mental patients turn to paperwork and concern with salaries and department of mental health functionaries turn to statistics and regulations, so mental health planners turn to fiddling with the system by changing the locus of care or funding arrangements. It does not work. We must return to the root problem of the patients and their care.

The Necessity of the Bureaucracy

The moment more than one person deals with something, one has "bureaucracy," in that it becomes necessary to have communication, consistency, and structure. At a certain critical point the organization becomes large enough so that these elements of the bureaucracy threaten to take on a life of their own, and rules, memoranda, and procedures begin to exist not to serve their original purpose (patient care) but to perpetuate their own existence (the bureaucracy). Governmental medicine, because of its task, cannot be regarded as cavalierly as the bureau of motor vehicles, and the bureaucracy must work to assist, not hamper, quality patient care.

Mental Health Desperately Needs a Constituency

To date, with the exception of a few crusading individuals (Dorothea Dix, Clifford Beers), concerned prominent citizens (Mary Lasker, Rosalynn Carter), and enterprising journalists (Albert Deutsch), there is not a strong consumer-based constituency to press for better care for the severely and chronically mentally ill. The powerlessness of both care givers and care receivers results in deplorable conditions and predictable scandals. Unless such a constituency develops among the general public, the adequacy of care of this population will depend on the whims of the legislators and their assessment of the needs of the patients rather than on an informed response to a well-organized and vocal group that can effectively present the needs of the severely and chronically mentally ill.

Changing Things for the Better Is difficult

Change processes are tricky in general, but in state hospitals they are almost impossible, since there are so many elements not subject to immediate understanding or manipulation. The only change that is feasible, given the complexity of the problems, seems to a systems one.

Systems Changes May Be the Beginning of a Solution

At its most conservative, a mental health systems change would have to pull together the disparate patchwork of elements in the system into a unified set of services. More radically, however, it might involve a system of vouchering or HMO's which would unify things not at the top but at the bottom, thus shaping the nature, location, and funding of services through consumer choice and option.

THEORETICAL ISSUES OF BROADER IMPORTANCE

This study of state mental hospitals has exposed several issues which relate to many more areas than that of mental health. As such, they are worthy of at least brief mention.

How a System Fails

The failure of the state mental hospital system provides a well-documented example of the failure of an entire social system to solve a problem for which it was designed. As such, it may provide analysts of social policy with an opportunity to examine the original objectives of the system, the planning of specific implementations to reach the objectives, the actual implementation carried out, the obstacles to realizing the intended objectives, and the maneuvers that a failing system goes through to maintain itself. For the most part, students of management and administration have limited themselves to individual organizations rather than entire industries, professions, or systems. It is important, however, to begin to examine the successes and failures of such larger systems, since we are inevitably moving toward their wider utilization.

The Problem with Government Running Human Services

As localities and regions have increasing difficulty managing large social problems, there is an increasing tendency to induce higher levels of government to assume funding and management of special services (e.g., welfare). Government, however, has a checkered career in the management of huge systems (e.g., the Postal Service, TVA, Veterans Administration), and it is unclear why its management works in some instances and not in others. If one merely limits this study to the health field, there is abundant data regarding the problems and potentials of both funding and directly managing health services. The state hospital system is an example where government has not covered itself with glory, and examining it versus the Public Health Hospital system, which has been largely successful, might provide some illuminating insights. These might help determine the future role of government in funding and managing future health services under national health insurance.

How Bureaucracies Work

Since Weber's initial exploration of the usefulness of bureaucratic structures,[1] there has been little serious attention paid to the issue mentioned in the previous section, that is, how bureaucratic structures assist or hamper the tasks of the organization. It seems clear that government and bureaucracies should exist to facilitate the implementation of society's goals. When the government or bureaucracy becomes more intent on preserving itself than on attaining its goals, it would seem to be counterproductive and worthy of study. Bureaucracies, like the jungle, are inherently neither good nor bad, but when they perform in an effective or destructive manner vis-à-vis their intended purpose, there is a necessity to examine the process and utilize the insights garnered. The state hospital system provides an ideal example of a system in which the bureaucracy's functioning is mostly counterproductive to its purpose and goals, and as such, it would be an ideal model for study.

Organizational Size as It Relates to Task

The problems in dealing with the severely and chronically mentally ill bring to the fore a question regarding whether large organizations can effectively deal with human services. It seems to me that the inherent value of increased size of an organization—e.g., increased efficiency, division of labor, ease of management, opportunity to purchase, plan and market in large masses, etc.—runs counter to the needs of providing an individual with human services, an enterprise that involves personal involvement, individual needs, specialized services, and attention to humanistic detail. In relation to mental health, it seems obvious that while funding may be creeping up the governmental ladder, service provision may necessarily be repositioned back at the most local level. Whether this is true of all human services remains to be seen, but it is an intriguing possibility that human services might function best when their funding is as distant and therefore politically invulnerable as possible, while their provision and implementation is as decentralized, local, and individualized as possible.

Centralization/Decentralization

A correlated issue concerns the relative centralization and decentralization of services. Certainly the pendulum has swung back most recently toward decentralization in education, police services, and industrial management, but there is always an argument concerning which services function better decentralized and which centralized. State hospitals and state hospital systems have also gone through several swings of the pendulum and are now moving toward decentralization along with other systems in society. Whether the residual central structure can diffuse itself outward after being compacted centrally is a question. Here again, the state hospital system could be a prime candidate for study.

Changing Organizations

The process of change and changing organizations represents an area of primary interest to a great number of individuals. To date, however, we lack a unified conceptual approach to change—one that is translatable into effective operational action in diverse fields. I would suspect that the change literature and change experiences in the mental health field are perhaps unique in their number and richness and could provide an abundant and diverse data base for further study.

The Defense Mechanisms of Social Institutions

Throughout this work reference has been made to the defensive maneuvers of individuals in the system to avoid the frustration of working with the difficult population served by the state hospital system. The adaptive and defensive maneuvers formed by the entire system to cope with its overwhelming problems have been identified and discussed in detail. This area, that of examination of the ways in which social institutions defend against problems of an overwhelming nature and struggle to maintain their equilibrium, is a fruitful one for investigation. The state hospital and the state hospital system once again would provide ample data for a study. As noted, there are abundant examples of the ways in which institutions struggle with, defend against, and adapt to complex problems, conflicting options, and difficult solutions.

CONCLUSIONS

The title of this work clearly implies that the mental health system is slowly moving toward the end of the state hospital and the death of the asylum. Whether and when this will happen depends on many variables, but that it will occur seems inevitable.

I suspect that there will continue to be attempts at cosmetic change of the state mental hospital system, primarily in terms of changes in its functioning and roles. The times and economic pressures, however, will force society to scrap the system eventually because of its inability to solve the tasks assigned to it, and we will see the end of the asylum. The death of the asylum will repeat history, however, in that it will not provide a solution to the problem—the treatment and care of the severely and chronically mentally ill. There will still need to be programs and services for this population—including asylumlike settings. Whether this needed system will arise phoenix-like out of the ashes of the asylum or replace it before its death is problematic.

In regard to the role of governmental psychiatry and medicine, I predict that we are moving inexorably toward a system of universal health coverage for some illnesses—but the problem of chronic and catastrophic diseases-may or may not be addressed by such coverage. I think this is a result of our social attitudes regarding both mental disorders and chronic diseases as well as the stigma of mental illness and the lack of an effective constituency for the severely and chronically mentally ill.

As for psychiatry, I think that the recent trend toward its remedicalization offers hope not only for the profession but also for the chronically ill mental patient—that is, if the profession does not abandon its role as advocate for these severely impaired individuals. As individual psychiatrists, we must deal with both the *reality* of treatment, care, and rehabilitation of the severely and chronically mentally ill, improving the technology, treatment resources, range, and number of services and studying comparative programs, as well as the *unreality* of governmental and bureaucratic defenses against dealing with the treatment of mental illness. Society will shuck off responsibility both for the state hospital system and the chronic mentally ill if given half a chance. We must not allow this to happen.

REFERENCE

1.   Weber, M: The Theory of Sound and Economic Organization. New York, Free Press, 1964 originally published in 1947

Index